# REFRESHING
# FOUNTAINS
## ON THE
# PILGRIMAGE

God bless you and thank you very much

# REFRESHING FOUNTAINS

# ON THE

# PILGRIMAGE

## HOW TO PROMOTE PSYCHOSPIRITUAL WELLNESS

**NDUNGU STEPHEN GITONGA (REV.)**

XULON PRESS

Xulon Press
2301 Lucien Way #415
Maitland, FL 32751
407.339.4217
www.xulonpress.com

Printed in the United States of America.
Edited by Xulon Press.

ISBN: 9781545608555

# DEDICATION

**This book is dedicated with a lot of love**
and devotion to the Most Holy Trinity, One God, for the marvelous work as stated in the opening of the Sacred Scripture: "In the beginning when God created the heavens and the earth . . . and found it very good" (Gen. 1:1, 31), (The Catholic Study Bible, 2nd ed). It is also dedicated to the Blessed Virgin Mary for her gentle accompaniment, and Holy Family of Jesus, Mary and Joseph, for their inspiration to families. To St. John Neumann, St. Francis, and St. Clare of Assisi, St. Stephen and all the saints for their constant intercession. To my dear parents, James and Mary Gitonga, and my siblings together with their families: P. Muciri and I. Irene, M. Jackson and F. Njoki, B.J. Muthoni (RIP) and M. Charles, M. Daniel and M. Wangari, M. Nyaguthii

and K. Simon, W.F. Rose and S. Mwaniki, S. Warukira and W. John, M. John and M. Muringi, and P. Warutumo. To my friends, relatives, teachers, neighbors, colleagues, and community for their great love, influence, and wisdom.

# ACKNOWLEDGMENTS

**With deep affection I acknowledge the** great love and support of many in all my life and ministry of which this work is a part. I am therefore first and foremost indebted to the church hierarchy and protocol: Pope Francis with whom I concelebrated a momentous mass he presided over for the world meeting of families in Philadelphia, 2015; Most Rev. Peter Kairo, Archbishop of Nyeri-Kenya for his fatherly accompaniment, and wise counsel, and for offering me chance for studies at Neumann University; Most Rev. Charles Chaput, Archbishop of Philadelphia for granting me residence, ministry, and generous provisions in the Archdiocese; Rev. Mons. D. Sullivan of the office for clergy in Philadelphia; Rev. J. Waweru, moderator of Nyeri, and Rev. P. Thamaini of Nyeri for their liaison for necessary protocols; And Rev. Efren V. Esmilla, the pastor of Our Lady of Hope for hosting me open-heartedly and to all parishioners, clergy, religious, and laity.

It is a pleasure to acknowledge with special gratitude Dr. Rosalie Mirenda, president of Neumann University, for supporting our archdiocese for advanced studies for clergy, religious, and laity, thus benefitting me in this benevolence and in her personal wise counsel. On same token I acknowledge Franciscan Sisters of Philadelphia, the founders of Neumann University. I also acknowledge great love and support from my family, relatives, and friends. I acknowledge the Neumann University community, along with the departments of Pastoral and Theological studies, Graduate studies, Library, International Students Office, and Mission and Ministry.

It would be an uphill task to attempt to list all involved in this work, but a few deserve special mention. Dr. L. DiPaolo Vice President of Neumann University Academic Affairs, Sr. M. Suzanne PhD, director of the Pastoral Counseling department, faculty members who taught me and those who supervised my field work: Dr. B. Toler, Dr. S. Park, C. Dougherty, G. Hall, Dr.

E. Flanagan, Dr. W. Fletcher, R. Douglas, Sr. T. Diane, PhD, Dr. J. Houck, Sr. M. O'Beirne, Rev. P. Lowe, Rev. S. Thorne, and Dr S. Lemon; the staff and students: Dr. D. Murphy, L. Kathryn, J. Mintzer, T. McGregor, Guillermo G., H. Jose, G. Daddona, G. Michelle, A. Rose, D. Bulinda, and F. Stephanie among others. I acknowledge the Belmont Behavior Hospital supervisors: R. Virginia, M. Scott, A. Rebecca, M. Dimario, and staff, patients and interns. I also acknowledge the Einstein Medical Hospital chaplaincy, staff, volunteers, and patients.

I acknowledge the Kenyan Catholic Community in America—clergy, religious, and laity: Rev. G. Muteru, Rev. S. Komu, Rev. J. Gathungu, Rev. R. Mwai, Rev. P. Kariuki, Rev. K. Martin, Sr. M. Muchire, Sr. M. Bakhita, the families of G. Marucha, G. Mbiu, D. Thiga, J. Kiarie, P. Wanjihia, F. Maina, C. Njeri, L. Waiganjo, J. Kiuna, D. Thuku, M. Dionisia, M. Mbugua, R. Ndeto, A. Mugo, A. Kirigwi, P. Mwangi, T. Katumbi, W. Carol, A. Mutinda, D. Ndegwa, M. Gituma, M. Mbatia, W. Munyao, and K. Catherine among others. Thanks to Sr. M. Helen, Sr. R. Rosa, Sr. M. Ann, Sr. N. Faith, Sr. Alice, Sr. Tony and the sisters of Mary Immaculate.

Special gratitude to Our Lady of Hope Parish community and families: Deacon H. Felipe, Deacon P. Homer, Deacon Rosario, Sr. M. Catherine, Sr. M. Loretta, Sr. B. Gertrude, J. Lopez, E. Gonzales,V. Fontanez, B. Evelyn, D. Miguel, P. Clark, I. Cruz, E. Monica, A. Stephens, R. Hill, J. Taimanglo, C. Brown, O. Thernell, B. Oakman, M. Matos, B. Turner, S. Josie, M. Patricia, H. Kossou, S. Anita, L. Mae, V. Salome, S. Mellisa, S. Suzzie, G. Euclides, , G. Maria, P. Rose, P. Lilian, D. Gregory, K. Stella, H. Naomi, J. Beverly, H. William, I. Palasol, C. Sayoc, C. Esmilla, T. Esmilla, and M. Ramcharan among others.

Colleagues in cultural ministry and across the United States deserve special mention: Rev. L. Bruce, Rev. Mons. H. Shields, Rev. Mons. R. Cheffo, Rev. L. Ogwochuku, Rev. L. Alfred, Rev. J. Okonski, Rev. G. Limbani, Rev. R. Landry, Rev. D. Roger, Rev. J. Muth, Rev. M. Francois, Rev. A. Nze, Rev. C. Walsh, Rev. R. Owens, Deacon B. Bradley, Deacon Mahoney, Sr. O. Florence, Sr. M. Clotilde, Sr. A. Lee, Sr. Kathleen, M. Davies, D. Harman, M. Ndicu, Dr. F. Tannian and G. Loretta among others. I also acknowledge colleagues in American Counseling

Association, American Association of Pastoral Counselors, Catholic Professionals—Archdiocese of Nyeri, Neumann University Alumni Association, Fairmount Park Conservancy, Knights of Columbus, and Knight of Peter Clavers.

I acknowledge enormous support from Nyeri Archdiocese and across Kenya, including clergy, religious, seminarians, novices, and laity. Among them I acknowledge H. E. John Cardinal Njue, Archbishop of Nairobi, Rt Rev. Bishop Philip Anyolo, Chairman of Kenya Catholic Conference of Bishops, Most Rev. Anthony Muheria, the New Archbishop of Nyeri, Rt Rev. P. Kihara, Rt Rev. K. Norman, Rt. Rev. M. Salesius, Rt Rev. W. James, Rt Rev. J. Obanyi, Very Rev. C. Kiruri, Vicar General of Nyeri, Rev. E. Gichuki, Rev. Prof. R. Wanjohi, Rev. E. Thuita, Rev. A. Mugi, Rev. J. Gichuki, Rev. J. Warui, Rev. P. Maina, Rev. J.B. Ndungu, Rev. J. Mwai, Rev. C. kinyua, Rev. E. Mutahi, Rev. N. Martin, Rev. S. Ngatia, Rev. I. Njogu, Rev. W. Theuri, Sr. M. Isaac, Sr. N. Magdaline, Sr. A. Kinya, Sr M. Kamara, Sr. A. Antonia, Sr. N. Nyambura, Sr. W. Jane, Sr. C. Njuguna, Br. G. Ouma, Br. J. Kamotho, R. Kiruki, P. Wangui, J. Waithaka, T. Kipkemoi, A. Mwihaki, M. Kihagi, J. Kaguru,

L. Muthoni, N. Lydia, and P. Njoroge among others. I also acknowledge the following parishes: Gatarakwa, Mugunda, Dundori, Manunga, Kahira-ini, Tetu, Kariko, Narumoru, Othaya, and Nyeri Consolata Cathedral.

I acknowledge with gratitude my pastors Rev. F. Romano and Rev. O. Elvino of Mugunda and Gatarakwa parishes along with clergy, religious, and laity, who hail from the region: Rev. M. Moses, Rev. J. Mbai, Rev. F. Mathenge, Rev. G. Ndung'u, Rev. P. Wachira, Sr. C. Gathigia, Sr. E. Kimani, Sr. L. Wangari, Sr. C. Wanjiru, C. Kimondo, S. Nderi, S. Kiriungi, B. Wanjiru, C. Wanjiku, J. Karu, T. Wambui, P. Mucemi, L. Nyawira, W. Rose, M. Wachira, G. Muthoni, J. Wambugu, M. Wangeci, G. Kiboi, and J. Maina, among many others.

I acknowledge St. Martin Catholic Social Apostolate Nyahururu, Kenya and their special ministry to the marginalized. I acknowledge Rt. Rev. L. Paiaro, Rt. Rev. J. Mbatia, Rev. G. Pipinato, Rev. J. Njoroge, Rev. P. Kimani, Rev. C. Muhindu, Sr. M. Mwangi, C. Ansram, K. Stephan, P. Ndogo, K. Joan, S. Maina, P. Ndiritu, R. Akoth, P. Kiruri, J. Baiye, Nasieku, Ngolong, Yasora, and K. Munderu.

Last but not least, special acknowledgments to R. Alicia for the secretarial consultation in manuscript compilation. W. Mary for manuscript review, encouragement, and publication financial support. Rev. G. Muteru for giving the foreword, brotherly accompaniment and generous support. And to Xulon Press for editing, typesetting, printing, and publication of this book, and you, dear esteemed reader, and all people of good will. God bless you!

# FOREWORD

**There is a deep rooted relatedness of all**
things. This relatedness has its primordial foundation in God
Himself who is a Trinity of Persons. The Three Persons of
the Trinity are one through love. This relatedness is also seen
between God and man for God is the origin and the point of
return for man who can only discover his true self in God. Man
is related to man and needs the others in order to discover his
true self. God in His perfection has emptied Himself to be man
so that man may discover him for his own good.

God has revealed Himself as a Trinity of persons that are
united into one by love. Everything tends to this unity of love
and oneness with God and with one another. The absence of
this relatedness and union causes anxiety where "the human

heart does not find rest until it rests in God". (St. Augustine, Confessions, Book 1, Chapter 1). The human person sets on a journey in search of this rest in terms of peace, tranquility and contentment in his life. Stephen Gitonga has described this journey as a pilgrimage where along the way man oscillates between search for God and for man either in family or in relationships or in therapy. He has tried to describe this journey in his book by using as analogy those he has met in his life and ministry who have embarked in the search for their self-discovery in vocation, relationships, work and career. He has continued on this journey too in his new found adventure as a pastoral counselor in attending his clients.

Through interaction with different people, some disturbed who are in need of healing, others sound of mind and body who would like to keep their sanity and others on the edge, the author finds a balance in the relatedness of all things that are in need of support along the way. Along the pilgrimage there is the healer and the one in need of healing, the counselor and the patient. This is a project that requires genuineness from the part of the healer as he calls the patient to self-discovery. The patient too has to walk the journey out of the bondage through the very difficult act of letting himself or herself be pulled out of the abyss of entanglement layer by layer of masks that have kept one (the patient) out of touch with his or her very self. With the aid of the counselor the patient has to discover his true self that lies there within that has been disfigured. Man reaches out to God and a boost from man helps man out of angst to self-discovery. The counselor walks the journey with the patient while trying not to impose his own will on the client by avoiding prejudicial attitude. He offers a road map as a guide along the way while keeping off the windshield to avoid becoming an obstacle himself. This enables the patient get a clear sight along the journey of self-discovery.

Stephen Gitonga has so well demonstrated in this book the relatedness that exists between man and man and his reaching out to God who is the culmination of the quest for self-discovery. This relatedness is not merely theoretical but practical. It is activated internally and externally where God and man are companions along the way of man's self-discovery. Stephen Gitonga in his book has tried to show that holistic healing requires man's discovery of himself through God. Man needs man for self-discovery (the patient needs the counselor) while God is the ultimate healer.

Rev. Gabriel Muteru, PhD.

Associate Professor, St. John University, Queens, New York.

# TABLE OF CONTENTS

# Chapter 1
## Introduction

**When it's thought to end or simply seems**
to end, it's actually just beginning. This thought, which characterizes our pattern of life and models our behavior, seems to find a deeper meaning as I reflect on my beginning of the program of Pastoral Clinical Mental Health Counseling rooted in Pastoral Care and Counseling at Neumann University. My interest in pursuing a deepened knowledge in counseling has a long history, dating back to early seminary days when I was sent for pastoral experience among communities as a young man and faced challenging questions about faith and life. Growing more mature and in the course of becoming a priest appointed to parish ministry, I then thought, *This is it; I know it all and*

*can now settle down and work.* However, the end became the beginning. Here I faced real issues requiring decisions, determinations, and direction for adults as well as the young. It is precisely in the work with young men, who are discerning their calling to priestly life and by extension, mission to young people and children in general, that vocation discernment propelled this inner desire for more. As the vocations director then and looking into the stories of these vocation aspirants, visiting their homes, and also facilitating seminars in schools for this respect, I felt now it was time to seek more training and acquire necessary competencies for deepened knowledge and skills in counseling ministry.

This long search characteristic of a journey was echoed in different voices by various clients I was privileged to work with, who oftentimes would say such words as: "I have been through a lot," "I realize things aren't the same,""I have lost something; I know not what but am here to begin the search,""I am here to work on my depression, addiction, . . .." or simply, "I don't know where to begin." As a pastoral counselor, I have come to know that this quest is not simply one way in the sense of the counselee seeking for direction, but it is a journey to travel together. This journey may take hours, days, weeks, months, or years. It prompts me to call it metaphorically a "Pilgrimage." Hunter (1990) defined *pilgrimage* as "a journey to a holy place . . . reasons for going on a pilgrimage are to receive healing from physical or emotional distress, to gain deepened religious insight . . . express thanksgiving to God . . ." (p. 923).

A person's life, too, in the context of counseling can be likened to a pilgrimage of wellness. This journey together has also deepened my ongoing self-discovery, especially as I ask myself the pertinent questions *Who am I? Where am I headed*, and *what are my resources to get there?* While answering these questions, I was quick to point out the enormous human resource at my disposal. The same is true of any other person asking him or herself these pertinent questions of life. The enormous human resources set before us at different levels serve as *Refreshing Fountains on the Pilgrimage.* On the journey, there will be times of getting weary, hungry, tearful, thirsty, angry, and distressed as was the case with the journey of Israelites from Egypt, crossing the Red Sea, and marching through the desert to Promised Land

(Ex. 14–17; Ps. 78). There will also be time to rejoice in hope as depicted by Israelites who, while not yet reaching the Promised Land and with other challenges awaiting them, nevertheless celebrated the victories of the moment. Even while pursued by Egyptian mighty army, they closed the Red Sea. And they "believed in the Lord and in Moses . . . sang this song . . . I will sing to the Lord, for he is gloriously triumphant" (Ex. 15:1ff.).

The journey with clients, like that of Israelites led by Moses (Ex. 14:10–31), Joshua (Jos. 3:1–17), Samuel (1Sam 3:19–21), and others, entails challenging moments at some point but always leads to celebrations of plausible successes along the way in large and small ways. As I set to present the feel of refreshing fountains on the pilgrimage, I note with delight those successful high points. I also acknowledge the challenging and low moments that point to near dead ends. Thanks are due to the enormous resources at disposal of clients and me in my role as therapist. The first of the resource is the person: inner strength, capacity to give and to receive, hopes, attitudes, beliefs, and values. I recently attended the sixty-fifth Annual Conference of American Counseling Association in San Francisco, California.

The key note speaker, Dr. Irvin D. Yalom, with a wide range of experience in clinical practice, constantly stressed client's inner resources that stand in need of exposition and exploitation for the benefit of the same client in therapy. Yalom (2002) earlier wrote on the client's share of responsibility in his or her own situation and more so in case of blame of another party in regard to one's difficult situation. He stated,

"Even if ninety-nine percent of the bad things that happen to you is someone else's fault, I want to look at the other one percent—the part that is your responsibility. We have to look at your role, even if it is very limited, because that is where I can be of most help" (p. 46).

The role of family, neighborhood, significant relations, school, job, and related human interactions are assets to be tapped. The sense of belief in God or higher power has its own special place. Other resources worth exploring include an enabling and empowering environment, safety, and caregiving. These resources, when well tapped, go a long way in wellness. They remind me of the biblical message: "a measure, packed together, shaken down and overflowing," (Lk. 6:38) as the lot from the Lord to his faithful people.

In all the above considerations, the person of the counselor stands to be in check. This cannot be done first and foremost by any other person apart from him or herself to begin with. Kornfeld (2012) gives a piece of advice to counselors as agents of wholeness, as she says, "you need to build into your weekly calendar time for your own self-care, personal and professional support, and continuing education." (p. 92). Caring for oneself is vital and cultivating this wholeness will impact on the wellness of others in this caring enterprise.

Important to self-care is self-awareness. Justes (2006) emphasizes the need for self-awareness as vital in counseling especially in relation to listening which is an essential counseling component. Justes says, "Primary in preparation for listening is self-awareness. Self-awareness, rigorously applied, helps spare us from listening disasters." (p. 21). To listen to others therefore calls to controlling of noises within ourselves which might be emanating from our previous experiences in family, classes, community, relationships, engagements and the list is endless.

Chapter 2
# Theological foundations

## Introduction

### The proclamation of sacred scripture in the

words, "O God come to my assistance" in the opening of Psalm
70:2 (New Jerusalem Bible, NJB) as often used in liturgical and
devotional church prayer has made a deep impression in my life
at various stages of my faith journey. In my priestly ministry
and given the fact that a priest is foremost a man of prayer, a
pleading with God on behalf of his people is inevitable:

> Every high priest is taken from among men and
> made their representative before God, to offer

gifts and sacrifices for sins. He is able to deal patiently with the ignorant and erring, for he himself is beset by weaknesses and so for this reason, must make sin offering for himself as well as for the people. No one takes this honor upon himself but only when called by God, just as Aaron was. (Heb. 5:1ff.).

A vivid description of my experience of this pleading with God for hastened assistance in a "can't wait" sort of attitude is in a pastoral engagement I undertook with children from the streets in my native Kenya. Assigned to an orphanage for children with many needs as part of my ministry, I soon realized the need for God's urgent intervention. While each was an individual, the story of each and every child was similar. The majority of the stories revolved around abandonment due to family constraints, breakups, HIV/Aids menaces, and other harsh conditions typical of slum living in suburban Kenya. These situations led to exposure of these children to all manner of abuse, including drugs, alcohol, trafficking, and prostitution.

Working with people in such situations as those of such children has been foundation for a journey of long search for purpose and destiny. At first I did not know where it would lead, but my pursuit of the program in pastoral counseling contributes to ongoing revelations for some parts of my spiritual journey. I imagine my experience as a search for refreshing fountains on the journey or "pilgrimage," which reminds me of the Samaritan woman who, having encountered Jesus, came to discover a fountain with living water within her. This discovery extended the conversation beyond bucket and water to a thirst quenched once and for all by the life-giving spirit of Jesus. She proudly exclaimed, "Sir, give me this water, so that I may not be thirsty or have to keep coming here" (John 4:15, NJB). The concept of Jesus as the one who quenches our thirst is depicted in Old Testament in the beautiful image of a thirsty deer. Only in God is our desire fulfilled as the Psalmist puts it, "As the deer longs for streams of water, so my soul longs for you, O God. My soul thirsts for God, the living God. When Can I enter and see the face of God?" (Ps. 42:2-3). In the New Testament, the same concept of Jesus quenching our thirst continues in different ways. A vivid capture of this quenching emerges thus, "let the one who thirsts come forward, and the one who wants it receive the gift of life-giving water" (Rev. 22:17). My wanting to pursue a path leading to the care of those in great need, and being a priest in service to all helps me understand more about universal call for all to ministry and even a further calling within a call for those especially prepared to such an undertaking. In this view I concur with the idea that,

> Pastoral counselors are often drawn to spiritual/ religious/theological education and the discipline of pastoral counseling in response to 'a call' in their lives, whether or not that call is understood to be from God or a transcendent source" (Snodgrass, 2015, p. 6).

Neumann University's comprehensive program in pastoral counseling has made me realize that much more work is needed on the part of each pastoral counselor to be in touch with his or her own being, core beliefs, and faith experience. A failure to be in tune with oneself risks his or her choosing short-cuts in attending and responding to people's needs.

Drawing on my experiences, first in Kenya and then in Neumann University, I am choosing to focus on three major perspectives that influence my theological foundations. They also involve the impact that comes from combining aspects of my experiences in the two worlds, namely the African and the American worldviews. My three core tenets include the family resilience in the light of the Holy Family, the loving relationship within the Trinity, and the importance of prayer in the context of the Word of God.

## The Holy Family and Resilience

The holy family of Jesus, Mary and Joseph, portrays a family in need, yet rich in all manner of possibilities for itself and for others. In the gospels the family of Nazareth emerges as one with few physical resources. Jesus was born in a manger, with parents in distress as expressed thus: "wrapped in swaddling clothes and laid him in a manger, because there was no

room for them in the inn" (Lk. 2:7). Even after his birth, Jesus'
family further endured many struggles (see Mt. 2:13; 2:14,
3:46). Yet, in this same family, we find a definitive outreach to
the community where they participate actively in the community affairs, as described in the context of wedding feast where
Jesus, following his mother's request, performs his first miracle
(John 2:1–12).

Growing up in a family of ten and by extension, large families on both maternal and paternal lineage prompted me to
espouse the theme of family and the diversity within each one.
Each member of any family brings around his or her unique-
ness despite some similarity in speech, behaviors, and attitudes.
This combination of difference and sameness invites a deeper
search of self and true identity. In my African background, I see
the root in which the family and community offers resources
upon which one draws to shape and enrich his or her own
identity. In the spiritual and religious sphere, this reality of my
family upbringing plays a major role. There were hardships in
our growing up, ranging from scarcity of food brought about
by repeated patterns of frequent droughts to a constant struggle

for access to clean water, healthcare facilities, better living conditions, and even basic education. In the efforts to make ends meet, religion, and with it spirituality, formed strength in my family. The hardships could have torn apart our family, but spirituality converged with the difficulties to breed resilience. Froma Walsh (2009), an original researcher on family resilience, articulates well what this means: "Family resilience involves key processes that enable the family system to rally in times of crisis: buffer stress, reduce the risk of dysfunction, and support optimal adaptation for all members."

Faithful endurance augments resilience well as Walsh (2009) further asserts, "Faith supports efforts to master the possible to accept that which is beyond control" (p. 42). The faith in God gives a special hope despite desperate situations. St Paul refers to such situation as "Hoping against hope" (Rom. 4:18) as he exemplifies trusting in God like Abraham did when he was tested to sacrifice his son of old age—despite the promise that he would become the father of a great nation through him.

In my work with clients, I quite often explore the family connection to find out some underlying strengths that may be untapped and which otherwise might be overlooked in turning around difficult situations toward opportunities for self-development. I remember a young adult client who shared on her need for pursuing higher studies but was finding herself at serious conflict with her mother. She also shared her feeling of disturbance over the absence of father figure in the house after her parents' divorce when she was younger, as well as the effect of household financial constraints. She constantly contemplated suicide or any other way of escaping from the stressful situation. In our sessions together, I gave her opportunities to explore more on her family situation and found out that the conflict was baffled more by other factors at play in the home. In addition to strained economics, there were also spiritual issues in which her different needs, including financial and religious independence as a growing young adult that were gradually emerging. In exploring these situations with her, she was able to gain insight into restating her goals, working toward them, and cultivating a better relationship with her mother. This led her to choose to continue her education. She began to realize why her mother was pushing her to do better and how she was making sacrifices with a constrained budget. This came as a wakeup call to her and led to her resolve for an amicable resolution to the conflict.

## The Trinity and Relationship

The image of a family joined together brings me to my second theme: that of the Trinity and the relationship within it that carries love, unity, and communion. This theme cuts across my core beliefs, and I cannot help employing it implicitly or explicitly in my clinical work. The Holy Trinity is understood as the unity of one God in three persons: Father, Son, and Holy Spirit (Mt. 28:19). This oneness is quite intricate, unfathomable, and mysterious; yet at the same time, attractive and desirable, so much so that each of the persons acts only in union with the others. Pope Francis in proclamation of the year 2016 as the Year of Mercy, offers us the understanding of God as Trinity from perspective of his closeness to us as he states, "With our eyes fixed on Jesus and his merciful gaze, we experience the love of the Most Holy Trinity. The mission Jesus received from the Father was that of revealing the mystery of divine love in its fullness." (cited in Kelly et al., 2015)

This idea of perfect unity is well articulated in Christ's promise of Pentecost. His words clearly show this Trinitarian communion as he says: "When the advocate comes whom I will send you from the Father, the Spirit of the truth that proceeds from the Father, he will testify to me" (Jn. 17).

The mysterious love of God is shared with humanity first in creation (Gen. 1:1) and especially creation of humankind "in his own image . . . male and female he created them" (Gen. 1:26, 27). Lartey (2003) expounds the Trinitarian love in his view of the intercultural pastoral care, emphatically stating that key is the realization that the love of God is for the whole world, created diverse and affirmed in its diversity by the creative energy of God. As such all that is done must respect and uphold the diversity in which the whole world is created (p. 30). The unconditional love of God, as Lartey (2003) describes it from the perspective of interculturality, further supports the Trinitarian formula of human personhood. Lartey (2003) explains that,

Every human person is in certain respects:

1. Like all others;

2. Like some others;

3. Like no other (p. 34).

These three statements underline the fact that we are all the same, and yet we are all different. Keeping this in mind as a pastoral counselor will help me approach each and every client as both other and no other. I will then see before me a person who hears, sees, thinks, feels, celebrates, or suffers in a unique way. From this understanding the common assertion, "I know how you feel," seems inappropriate if not dangerous when quickly applied to another person's experience without due care.

Jesus Christ's love and closeness to us is a revelation of the indwelling Trinity within us. It is very thrilling to discover how special revelation of Jesus in our journey brings joy and contentment. This reminds me of the Emmaus episode in the Bible when two disciples had a special encounter with Jesus on their journey that transformed their lives. This transformation not only restored their waning hope, but provided true joy to the extent that they recalled the feelings deep within their hearts and, thrilled with this joy, shared the story to encourage their brethren. They said, "Were not our hearts burning (within us) while he spoke to us on the way and opened the scripture to us?" (Lk. 24:32).

## Prayer and Meditation on the Word of God

The third theme of my core beliefs treated in this chapter is prayer and meditation on Word of God. My experience of prayer and meditation on God's Word goes hand in hand with my ministry as a priest. A priest is essentially meant to be a man of prayer and meditation on the Word of God after the pattern and manner of Jesus Christ, the high priest. Jesus Christ is the same yesterday, today, and forever (Heb. 13:8). He is the Word that was in the beginning with God, and the Word was God. (Jn. 1:1–3). After his resurrection, Jesus explained to the disciples going from Jerusalem to Emmaus all that was written about him in all the scriptures beginning with Moses and all the prophets (Lk. 24:25–27). The entire scripture therefore relates to him and is summarized in him, for it tells about him, and through him the triune God is revealed: God the Father and the Son and the Holy Spirit. We draw from Jesus a great parallel on the importance of unity between Old and New Testament that is evident in his teaching on prayer, precisely the prayer of our Father (Lk. 11:2–4; Mt. 6:9–13). As Pope Benedict xvi (2006) notes:

> Our Father, then, like the Ten Commandments (Ex. 20: 1ff, Deut 5:6ff.) begins by establishing the primacy of God, which then leads naturally to a consideration of the right way of being human . . . Nothing can turn out right if our relation to God is not rightly ordered. For this reason, the Our Father begins with God and then, from that starting point, shows us the way toward being human (p. 134).

The priestly prayer of Jesus (Jn. 17) teaches us a lot about prayer to God and its connection with his Word that he is (Word made flesh, Jn. 1:14). He says to his disciples:

> "But now I am going to the one who sent me . . . for if I do not go the Advocate will not come to you . . . But when he comes, the Spirit of truth, he will guide you to all truth . . . He will glorify me, because he will take from what is mine and declare it to you. Everything that the Father has is mine; for this reason I told you that he will take from what is mine and declare it to you" (Jn. 16:5–15).

This experience of prayer to me is rooted in recited family prayers and devotions, such as daily recitation of the rosary, singing sacred songs, and constant reading of the Bible and of the lives of saints while growing up. Such was the power of prayerful environment that gave us hope amidst hopelessness and resonates with what St. Paul refers to as "hoping against hope" (Rom. 4:18). I remember clearly the daily recitation of the rosary by the family after the dinner around the fire place and before retiring to bed. The prayer took the form of a tune which you would at times murmur halfway asleep in our childhood, in a manner suggesting, "when will I get out of here?" However, it was a rule that we had to abide by and our mother was keen to make everyone awake and attentive. I still hear that music of the rosary tune in mind from time to time.

Today prayer with Bible reading and meditation is still central in my daily routine and now with much more fervor and deeper meaning than obligation back in the day in my upbringing. Prayer for me incorporates responsibility for others, and in this I concur with St. Theresa of the Child Jesus. A biographer of hers states: "Theresa does not cease to hear this prayer of God which speaks to her of her responsibility toward every being" (Six, 1998, p. 178). With Theresa I have come to see the journey of prayer as a journey of faith like that of the Israelites as narrated in Sacred Scriptures which constitutes advancement or progression in stages. Echoing the faith development work of Fowler (2000), the work of growing is never done: "The crucial point to be grasped is that the image of human comple-tion or wholeness offered by faith development theory is not an estate to be attained or a stage to be realized. Rather it is a way of being and moving, a way of being on pilgrimage" (p. 60).

The growth I continually seek in prayer is at times not noticeable. At those times I must dispose myself to stay with the reality of unknown, trusting thus like a sower: "It is as if a man were to scatter seed on the land and would sleep and rise night and day and the seed would sprout and grow, he knows not how" (Mk. 4:26). A deepening of knowledge in my spirituality and theology gives me a background to engage in understanding religious faith tradition as that which influences consciously or unconsciously my way of being. This is captured in the sense of an ongoing story: "Understanding religiousness and spirituality as a sacred narrative is a unique quality of pastoral assessment and enormously advantageous for understanding the religious and spiritual worlds in which clients dwell" (Deal and Magyar-Russell, 2015, p. 121).

In the terms of clinical work performed in my pastoral role, I have experienced times when clients sought divine intervention, precisely in asking for special prayers and also biblical verses and oftentimes the whole Bible. In these encounters, such phrases are common: "Can you say a prayer for me?" "What verse of the Bible can encourage me when depressed?" and "Please, remember my loved ones in your prayer." These prayer requests are more frequent when I meet with clients who recognize me as a priest. More often the client will say, for instance, that he or she needs lots of prayers in his or her addiction, for surgery, or simply in general terms for a home situation. These prayer requests have been the entry points for me to engage the spiritual aspect in the person from my pastoral counseling disposition. In this sense, prayer becomes an experience of thirst in a two-fold manner as expressed in the story of Jesus and the Samaritan woman. The first is the expressed "unimaginable" thirst of Jesus in the sense of pleading for a drink while in the actual sense he is yearning for the redemption of this woman. The other kind of thirst is the unexpressed one by Samaritan woman, which is obvious for every Christian, and that is the thirst for Jesus. The encounter of Jesus with the Samaritan woman reveals this two-fold thirst that goes so far beyond the bucket and the well (Jn. 4:1ff.).

The image that I have for a pastoral counselor is shaped to a great extent by this idea of Jesus' thirsting for souls, so much so that at his death he expresses the depth of his love by saying, "I thirst" (John 19:28). I envision a pastoral counseling ministry in which the counselor journeys with the client to the point of discovery that both of them knows their thirst quenched by him, who is able to know even beyond the counselor's and client's limits. In this episode, each person can come to Jesus and embrace their vulnerability like that of Samaritan woman in seeking to fulfill his or her thirst. The process becomes a sign of great communion.

The searching for what does quench spiritual thirst is not only a joy for the two pilgrims, but as Fowler (2000) envisages the growth of faith, it is "a way of being and moving, a way of being on pilgrimage" (p. 60). But this journey is also a confirmation of the transformative nature of the process in which the counselor and client are only agents. Prayer therefore as a communication between God and his people as traditionally held is also, as St. Theresa calls it, a triumph of love "which stooping over the nothingness, transforms it into love" (Six, 1998, p. 85). In this way, God, whose wisdom is beyond limit and who is never outdone in goodness, in a special way discerns the desire of the believer and in magnanimity grants forgiveness and consoles a heart that prays in trust, as Jesus promises, "Your heavenly Father knows you need them all" (Mt. 6:8-32; Lk. 12:29–32). A life of prayer is a reflection of the unconditional love that compels us to embrace all others in the same way our heavenly Father does (1 John 4:7–8; John 13:34–35).

The scripture cements our prayer following the pattern of Jesus and many other biblical figures who put their total trust in God and were never disappointed. These were such as Abraham in the great test of sacrificing his son Isaac (Gen. 22:9–14), Hannah and the birth of Samuel (1 Sam. 1:9ff.) and Daniel in the lion's den (Dan. 6:16ff.). A summary of prayer and meditation on the Word of God is perfectly captured in Israelites' great prayer beginning thus: "Hear O, Israel" (in Hebrew, known by those very opening words–*shema yisra'el*):

Hear O Israel! The Lord is our God the lord alone! Therefore, you shall love the Lord, your God with your whole heart, and with your whole being, and with your whole strength. Take to heart these words which I command you today. Keep repeating them to your children. Recite them when you are at home and when you are away, when you lie down and when you get up. Bind them on your arm as a sign and let them be as a pendant on your forehead. Write them on the doorposts of your houses and on your gates (Dt. 6:4–9).

The relationship of prayer and meditation on the Word of God can be summed in the Christian tradition called "Lectio Divina," or praying the scriptures. Dr. Houck, a professor of pastoral counseling in Neumann University, who is also a church minister and a prolific writer, articulates best what Lectio Divina means:

With lectio divina, scripture is read slowly, attentively, reflecting on a single word or phrase that may be God's instruction for us. The more we engage in this type of scriptural reflection, the more we discover how much we are able to open ourselves to an ever intimate relationship with God, becoming more attuned to the Holy Spirit's presence in our lives (Houck, 2009 p. xviii).

The more we pray with scriptures, the more we grow in depth of knowledge of God and ultimately in union with him. Merton Thomas (1971) stresses:

The spiritual understanding of scripture leads to a mystical awareness of the Spirit of God himself living and working in our own souls, carrying out by His mysterious power, in our own lives, the same salvific actions which we

27

can see prefigured and then realized in the Old and New Testaments (p. 29).

Prayer to God continues to offer sense of safety, confidence and protection. The psalmist puts it clearly saying, "So let each faithful pray in the time of need. The floods of water may reach high but such a one they shall not reach." (Ps. 32:6).

## Conclusion

The expression of the spiritual and theological foundation of my pastoral identity resonates with Franciscan view of love and self-giving to God and his people. St. Francis of Assisi cooperated in strenuous ways to exemplify through his life this love and providence of God to humanity. This is especially so in his prayer, belief in God, and sense of "extended family," namely the vulnerable, poor, and needy. This is evidenced by many writings and witnesses about him in form of prayers, songs, and poetry. An example of this follows as expressed thus:

From the granary of poverty

Saint Francis drew supplies to feed

The famished throng that followed Christ,

Lest on their journey they grow weak.

The road to glory he spreads out,

Enlarged the way that leads to life.

For being poor in this world's goods

He reigns rich in his true homeland,

And constitutes his kingly heirs

Those poverty on earth enriched."

(Julian of Speyer (1999), The Divine Office of

St. Francis)

# Chapter 3
# Psychological foundations

## Introduction

### A new client presented himself in a group

that I was leading as an intern in a mental health hospital. The client's entry in the group was characterized by anxiety, withdrawal, flat affect, confusion, and frustration. This client sat in a corner facing the wall and upon being prompted to participate would turn briefly and then face the wall again. I tried to redirect him to the group activity to no avail. At the end of the group, I invited him to an individual meeting just to check with him on what was going on and what was it that I could do to encourage him to participate or help him process the feelings of the moment. He sat facing me and paused for some time. The feelings going on within me were that he was having a bad day or that in his condition he was not able to talk to strangers as someone just new in the facility.

I could feel myself becoming concerned and started to prompt him to speak. He finally sat back and, looking at me, said, "I hate the activity of meditation you began with." I asked him to share more about this and what else he liked or disliked in the group, and to my amazement he said he was following everything. Wanting to test this, I asked him a couple of things that transpired in the group, and he accurately pointed them out. He further said that he did not want to face some people in the group who looked like people who cause trouble in his neighborhood. I noticed some relationship dynamic at play in this encounter and took advantage of this unfolding to build an environment of safety and freedom. I can identify the whole of this encounter as being very Rogerian, as I will explore in this chapter.

In the course of my learning and clinical work with cli-ents I have come to identify with person-centered or Rogerian relational and interpersonal dynamics of psychotherapy. In the heart of this theory is Rogers's (Carl Ransom Rogers, 1902-1987) notion of the "helping relationship." This term, helping relationship, in Rogers's conception emerges as he articulates it:

> My interest in psychotherapy has brought in me an interest in every kind of helping relationship. By this term I mean a relationship in which at least one of the parties has the intent of promoting the growth, development, maturity, improved functioning, improved coping with life of the other. The other in this sense may be one individual or a group. To put in another way, a helping relationship might be defined as one in which one of the participants intends that there should come about, in one or both parties, more appreciation of, more expression of, more functional use of the latent inner resources of the individual" (Rogers, 1961, p. 39).

This definition of a helping relationship, as Rogers views it, fits a wide range of relationships that intend to facilitate growth such as those between mother and child, physician and patient, teacher and pupil, and counselor-client relationships. He (1961) further explores the wide range of counselor-client relationships:

> such as between psychotherapist and the hospitalized psychotic, the therapist and the troubled or neurotic individual, and the relationship between the therapist and the increasing number of so called "normal" individuals who enter therapy to improve their own functioning or accelerate their personal growth. (p. 40)

In looking through Rogers's approach in person-centered therapy, along with my encounters with various clients with different personal needs, attitudes, reactions, and temperaments in my clinical work, I find a great deal of resonance leading to my orientation to the choice and application of this therapy.

This is particularly true in reference to recognition of each client's inner potential that can be called out or harnessed through this helping relationship. As Rogers emphasizes, through the counseling relationship "there should come about, in one or both parties, more appreciation of, more expression of, more functional use of the latent inner resources of the individual" (Rogers, 1961, p. 40). As depicted by the client earlier cited as closed in the group though later opens up in the individual encounter, building relationship is facilitated when the client can be the expert. A conviction I have come to espouse is that the client has inner strengths capable of developing to full potential given necessary conditions. These necessary conditions strive to give the client the power lost in course of subjective experiences—relational and systemic dynamics. In this way the client is able to place him or herself back to the path of self-discovery and hence engage in self-actualization. This idea gives the core of Rogers's teaching on the principle of self-actualization. Rejecting the determinism that was prevalent in other theories, particularly behaviorism and psychoanalytic, Rogers (1951) insisted that "The organism has one basic tendency and striving—to actualize, maintain, and enhance the experiencing organism" (p. 487).

Having explored Rogers' person-centered approach and indeed other existential-humanistic approaches to therapy in which this approach is rooted, I have come to identify with some of the core characteristics and elements involved therein. These are summarized in Rogers's (1957) hypothesis of the six core conditions which he argues are based on many years of his professional experience in the person-centered theoretical approach. Rogers in this view therefore emphasizes that,

For constructive personality change to occur, it is necessary that these conditions exist and continue over a period of time. These core conditions are:

1.  Two persons are in psychological contact.
2.  The first, whom we shall term the client, is in a state of incongruence, being vulnerable or anxious.
3.  The second person, whom we shall term the therapist, is congruent or integrated in the relationship.
4.  The therapist experiences unconditional positive regard for the client.

5. The therapist experiences an empathic understanding of the client's internal frame of reference and endeavors to communicate this experience to the client.

6. The communication to the client of the therapist's empathic understanding and unconditional positive regard is to a minimal degree achieved (p. 95).

The core conditions Rogers provides are necessary for change and growth in the client and therapist's journey together. They stem from the central hypothesis which Rogers (1980) postulates that, "Individuals have within themselves vast resources for self-understanding and for altering their self-concepts, basic attitudes, and self-directed behavior; these resources can be tapped if a definable climate of facilitative psychological attitudes can be provided" (p. 115). I have come to identify with many elements within the six core conditions necessary for self-growth in Rogers' hypothesis, both personally and therapeutically as a counselor. The three main elements among many others that have resonated with my training and practice as a pastoral counselor, as well as enhancing my current engagement as a church minister, include those of relationship, self-discovery for self-actualization, and active listening.

## Therapeutic Relationship

As I explore the element of relationship, what comes to mind are the daily interactions I make with different people in different planes, be it in family, business, or otherwise. My experience attests to the poetic line that "No man is an island." Through my experience of such interactions at Neumann University, I have acquired a great deal of learning and an appreciation particularly of American culture while also sharing my experience of African culture within a listening, honoring, and caring relationship. From an African view, for instance, community spirit permeates family and individual spheres to a great extent. A dysfunctional family as is the case with a dysfunctional individual in this sense is viewed as a community's responsibility to address. Seeing relationships through the lens of Rogers' principle of the helping relationship has helped me understand what distinguishes real relationship, especially in the sense of people being heard or understood. I am drawn to three main components of this relationship, based on Rogers' six core conditions while attending to clients, namely genuineness, unconditional positive regard, and empathic understanding. The unconditional positive regard in a way encompasses these others, and therefore its exemplification touches on them, too.

Unconditional positive regard, according to Rogers (1980), is also referred to as acceptance, caring, or prizing (valuing with high esteem). In this the therapist accepts each individual and lets the client be who he or she is in the moment and experience—"whatever immediate feeling is going on—confusion, resentment, fear, anger, courage, love, or pride" (p.116). The same case of caring for an individual in a one-on-one encounter in such a way that he or she feels and presents his or her authentic self is true of an individual in group. Rogers (1970) says:

> I am centered in the group member who is
> speaking ... I want him to feel from the first that
> if he risks saying something highly personal, or

absurd, or hostile, or cynical, there will be at least one person in the circle who respects him enough to hear him clearly and listen to that statement as an authentic expression of himself (p. 47).

To provide such a condition of safety, the therapist needs to work on his or her own issues, which may stand in the way of this condition of relationship. This includes addressing some of the prejudices that might be at play in his or her own world, including those of race, ethnicity, sex, religion, experience, temperament, education, and culture.

There are a few times when I find myself holding some opinions or stereotypes regarding certain people based on the aforementioned categories of race, religion, and ethnicity. Sometimes what I feel may spill over onto my clients if they belong to such populations. To keep this in check on my part, I have been involved in personal therapy and supervision. I also continue studies in personal growth and awareness as well as being mindful of areas of personal limitations in order to make necessary improvements. Unconditional positive regard, therefore, has played a key role in nurturing my experience. I appreciate Rogers (1957), who wrote, "It means a caring for the client, but not in a possessive way or in such a way as simply to satisfy the therapist's own needs. It means a caring for the client as a separate person, with permission to have his own feelings, his own experiences." (p. 98).

## Self-Discovery for Self-actualization

The ancient recommendation "to know thyself" is central, especially in discerning what move one ought to make in pursuit of self-goals in life. This self-discovery is never a one-time event but one which is comprised of billions of steps toward a final destination of the highest sense of self-actualization. In my work with clients, I constantly encounter questions of connection to self and life, which ultimately comprises other complex questions. My pondering this has always presented itself in one way or the other, and when it does, I find it worth considering as a matter of urgency. I recall some clients who at various times pose questions to me such as: "What am I going to do about my addiction? About my spiritual search? About my failing relationship?" Rogers (1961) points out the move toward the direction of self-discovery and self-actualization by exploring each client's unique experiences. This he succinctly captures as:

> Below the level of the problem situation about which the individual is complaining- behind the trouble with studies, or wife, or employer, or with his own uncontrollable or bizarre behavior, or with his frightening feelings, lies one central search. It seems to me that at bottom each person is asking, 'Who am I, really? How can I get in touch with this real self, underlying all my surface behavior? How can I become myself? (p. 108).

What prevents most of the people from self-discovery and, therefore, from a movement to self-actualization is the existence of a façade. Clients' façades, as Rogers (1961) refers to them, are "the false fronts, or the masks, or the roles with which one has faced life" (p. 109). In struggling to discover one's true self, many insights present themselves, though this entails a long and painstaking journey. Rogers (1961) points out the inner satisfaction and reward after overcoming the problem of the façade as he states: "To remove a mask which you had thought was part of your real self can be deeply disturbing experience; yet, when there is freedom to think and feel and be, the individual moves toward such a goal" (p.110).The use of this Rogerian concept of self-discovery has yielded in me a deep sense of satisfaction. In the session, I find myself sitting back reflectively with clients, especially at their deepest moments of life struggles. In this path into self-discovery, I have seen clients peel off layer after layer of defenses, or "masks," and gradually sinking into the "aha" of the person who lies beneath and who now begins to confidently emerge, precisely as the true self. The true self, therefore, can take control of a person's life and with freedom direct it to desirable end, which, in the case of so many of clients, can be referred to as self-actualization.

## Active Listening

Another key aspect in Rogerian person-centered therapy is active listening; in fact, it might be called the hallmark of Rogerian therapy. In an article titled "Active Listening," (Roger and Farson, 1987) state that "Clinical and research evidence clearly shows that sensitive listening is a most effective agent for individual personality change and group development" (p. 1). The article further enumerates important components of listening, which range from how to listen, the do's and don'ts, what is communicated in listening, and even to considering the problems of active listening. It is quite fascinating to discover how this ordinary activity of listening has far-reaching consequences, whether negative or positive, and has so often influenced the world. A case in point is where some politicians or influential leaders in societies say something today and deny the same tomorrow. Some pronouncements with less reflection or listening to the self in this scenario have even incited hearers or led to gross misunderstandings that have wreaked havoc. When the listener is in tune with the speaker and thus is exhibiting effective listening skills, including interest and curiosity, the speaker tends to pick up on the interest and becomes more captivated to articulate the message and even go deeper. The inverse is also true; loss of interest in the speaker leads to loss of the message and can consequently make the speaker shut down or present an inauthentic message, communicated just for its own sake. In a world filled with numerous cares with minimal time it is a risky or painstaking business to listen to someone to the extent that the individual feels understood.

To hold the other person's point of view and hold one's own view is not easy. It is enhanced when the therapist is willing and able to show interest in the speaker (client) so as to listen attentively to him or her, and thus be able to see the world as the client does or rather experience it from his or her standpoint. This kind of listening cannot come about without certain dispositions involving attending, which, as explored earlier, ties to the quality relationship in a broader sense. In trying to understand the client, Rogers (1961) offers his own experience of when a person comes to him, as he shares, "It is my purpose to understand the way he feels in his own inner world, to accept him as he is. To create an atmosphere of freedom in which he can move in his thinking and feeling and being, in any direction he desires." (p. 108).

This explanation of Rogers on striving to understand the client brings in an aspect of openness in active listening that entails more than just verbal and nonverbal communication in the session. The importance of active listening places a demand of self-discipline on the part of the therapist to be in control of his or her inner and outer subjective experiences to a high degree, lest a spill from either of these alters the client's path to change and wholeness.

I recall one day having received the news of the demise of my grandmother, and later in the week having a crucial appointment with a client who had been struggling with grieving the loss of her son. I took substantial time to process my loss, including sharing with my colleague priests, and as the appointment neared, I kept reminding myself that it's not about me and my experience at the moment but about providing a listening ear to my client. The session went on well to my amazement with moments of empathic understanding standing out, especially with some recourse to our common practice of Christian faith. As I sat listening actively to the client's sharing, the biblical image that ran across my mind, which also benefitted me in the moment, was 2 Corinthians 1:3–4: "Blessed be the God and Father of our Lord Jesus Christ, . . . who encourages us in our every affliction so that we may be able to encourage those who are in any affliction." Another image that was coming to my mind is one that I remember sharing with my professor, and that was the image of crossing guard meeting a client at a certain point and a certain juncture in their lives; in this case at an intersection, the therapist watches the person do the actual crossing at that juncture and then confidently proceeds on their own with the rest of the journey. Of interest is that implication of meeting the client at an intersection—at a particular point and juncture in someone's life.

I have come to understand that, as the counselor, I can cultivate active listening by first learning to pay attention to the self-picture I hold of myself. In this self-picture, the counselor needs to constantly take cognizance of growing edges or limitations and work in the direction of addressing them, while at the same time, enhancing his strengths so that he or she may be always authentically effective. When I looked back to how I have listened to myself in the past, I came to discover how much more I needed to do the real listening. This realization quickly put me on the path of intentionally listening to myself, using various techniques such as mindfulness, deep breathing, and using each of my five senses for self-awareness. Using these techniques, I have learned to take note of what is going on in my mind in the moment and what it is that I need to do.

I remember a client who I journeyed with in his struggle with alcoholism. In his initial encounter, this client stated that he was fed up with himself and he had reached his end. He further went on to say that he felt lonely and just closed himself in the house and drank himself to death. In his own words, he said, "Not one, not two days but uncountable, while drinking I forgot everything else, including who I am or where I am." I attended to him in Rogerian active-listening technique, which led him to go deeper, and in the course of many sessions, he was able to discover many other things that he had never felt courageous to share and which he discovered were taking toll on his life and thus contributing to an escalating drinking problem. This discovery I would attribute it to the active listening offered him in the meeting space where even such nonverbal messages like tears and facial expressions were received in the wider context and reflected back to him therapeutically in the words, "I hear you."

Letting the client engage with him or herself and with the therapist, who is there to listen and reflect with the client, produces tremendous effect on positive change. The therapist's goal, therefore, is to listen for total meaning, that is, the message and the feelings behind the message. In this area of listening, I see my goal as first reflecting back the client's previous point before jumping on to the next point so as to ensure that I understand clearly. At the same time this repetition can help the client clarify his or her train of thought with an assurance that he or she is being heard. Again, Rogers (1981) emphasizes this idea of active listening or "hearing the client" as he observes:

> When I truly hear a person and the meanings that
> are important to him at that moment, hearing

not simply his words but him and when I let him

know that I have heard his own private personal

meanings, many things happen. There is first of

all a grateful look. He feels released. He wants

to tell me about his world. He surges forth in a

new sense of freedom. He becomes more open

to the process of change (p. 116).

## Conclusion

Rogers's person-centered theory that has influenced my

practice of pastoral counseling has not only laid emphasis on

the six core constructs necessary for creating the necessary

climate of change. It has expounded on other elements in my

general framework of counseling. Some of these elements and

the three tenets that I already have discovered and built upon

include therapeutic relationship, self-discovery for self-ac-

tualization, and active listening. The quality of listening, for

instance, is not only useful in counseling, but is also a quality

able to permeate all my facets of relationships with others.

Lack of clarity in communication in the face of the contemporary information explosion can lead to misunderstanding and extensive damage to relationships. All these key characteristics, collectively considered, weave and warp together for a unified whole.

At the end of his life, Rogers was recognized for what his theory could contribute to this unified whole. He himself (1980) enumerated some of its impact, stating that ". . . studies have been made of the benefits of person centered psychotherapy with troubled individuals and with schizophrenics; of facilitation of learning in the schools; of improvement in other interpersonal relationships" (p. 117). As I consider the impact of this theory, I find it worthwhile for person-centered theory forming a strong foundation upon which my pastoral counseling rests, even when employing other techniques and elements. May I, like Rogers, always keep in mind and heart the client's best interests and needs.

# Chapter 4
# Clinical Case Presentation

## I. Service Rendered

90834 Psychotherapy, 45 minutes with the patient

## II. Client Identifying Information

D is a 45-year-old Caucasian female. She is single and has never been married. She is a Baptist Christian who holds a high school diploma.

## III. Personal History

A. **Psychosocial/Developmental History**

**D is one of six children, four brothers and** one sister. D has a son, aged 26 years. Her parents are both living but divorced. The mother lives with D's aunt. D reports having a challenging upbringing; she was particularly slow-learning, which led to her being looked down on by the parents, siblings, and peers. She reports suffering rejection right at childhood and was referred to as "stupid "and even "retarded." She reports a series of incidents of sexual abuse at childhood. She also reports being molested by her cousin between the ages of 11 and 15, as well as being raped by a different party at age 12.

D reports that her mother, her younger brother, and her son, suffer from depression similar to hers. D reports that apart from that rejection at childhood, the family has been relating well with her, especially nowadays. She reports that she has a strong bond with herfather and mother despite their being divorced. D reports that her depression kicked in at her early 20s. At the age of 24, D recalls using marijuana 2–3 times a day. She states she has been admitted to several hospitals for depression. In January 2015, D reports having suicidal ideations and behavior of cutting herself with a paper clip. She describes feeling helpless, useless, and worthless and thus often thinks of suicide.

D reports that she has been hospitalized in the current facility for the second time this year for depression and suicidal ideations. She reports having tried to suffocate herself with a towel once in the current facility, and several times she has been scratching and cutting herself with her nails.

## B. Substance Abuse History

D reports using Marijuana from age 24 until her admission as inpatient in this facility in March 2015.She reports having used the substance 2–3 times a day.

## C. Medical History

D has Diabetes mellitus, type 2; mixed hyperlipidemia; gastroesophageal reflex disease (GERD); asthma; high blood pressure; morbid obesity; and iron deficiency.

# IV. Past Psychiatric Treatment

## A. Past Mental Health Treatment

D reports being hospitalized in a facility for the first time in 1997 at age 27 for depression. Since then she has regularly been seeing an outpatient psychiatrist who has been monitoring her progress.

D has also had multiple in-patient admissions in various hospitals and facilities. She has also had ECT (electroconvulsive therapy) and EMDR (eye movement desensitization and reprocessing) treatments.

## B. Past Psychiatric Meds

D reports using some medicines for her depression and is complying accordingly. Some of the meds she has used include lithium duloxetine 300 mg daily for anxiety control, trazodone for depression and anxiety, and Zoloft for depression.

## C. Past Psychiatric Diagnosis

D has been diagnosed in the past with Major depressive disorder with psychotic features, 296.34 (F.33.3); Borderline personality disorder 301.83 (F.60.3) and Schizophrenia 295.90 (F20.9)

## V. Current Encounter.

### A. Overall Chief Complaint/Presenting issue

D's overall complaints are "I am a little bit upset" and "They moved my unit, and I hate change." D says she is upset by a peer whom she dislikes as a roommate. She also says she has another peer who upsets her in the unit, though not in the same room. D says that her unit was merged with another one, and they moved to that other unit. She says that this change of unit has affected her mood (being upset).

### B. History of Present Condition/Illness

D says that she feels worthless and helpless most of the time. She feels that she needs someone to share with about her problems. She says that her family has mental health illnesses, too (mother, brother, and son have depression), and she does not want to bother them. She says that sometimes thoughts about her past are overwhelming and upsetting, especially childhood sexual and verbal abuses. She admits that she has been experiencing disturbing flashbacks and nightmares and racing thoughts, which are sometimes out of her control.

She blames herself for everything happening to her and her family. She blames herself for the rape at age 12, saying that she should have prevented it because she knew what was right or wrong. She also blames herself for being upset with peers, stating that she is always on the wrong side. She says that she hates change, and any change aggravates her suicidal thoughts. This makes her more upset and depressed. She also says that she feels lonely and depressed due to the long hospitalization (11 months) in the current facility.

## C. Review of Current Psychological Symptoms

D perceives herself as helpless and with limited choices. She is frustrated by events of her past and carries the blame and guilt with her all the time. She blames herself for all wrong or failure happening around her. D has limited insight into the progress she is making in spiritual, physical, and mental wellness exercises. D feels lonely and helpless. She feels the need to do what she is supposed to do but lacks the courage to begin and sustain it on the account of fear of failure. She feels tired of living and listens to the negative voices telling her she is a failure or to end her life.

## D. Mental Status

| | |
|---|---|
| Appearance: | tidy, hair well done |
| Attitude: | cooperative, though anxious |
| Motor Activity: | still |
| Speech: | normal, paused |
| Affect: | flat |
| Mood: | anxious |
| Thought Process: | interrupted, irrational |
| Thought Content: | coherent |
| Presence of Hallucinations: | yes (hearing voices) |
| Suicide Ideations: | yes |
| Homicidal Ideations: | none reported |
| Presence of Delusions: | yes |
| Memory: | intact |
| Self-Perception: | distorted, low self-esteem |
| Judgment: | limited |
| Insight: | limited |
| Orientation to Time, Place, Person: | x3 |

### E. ASSESSMENT/DSM 5 Diagnosis

## Initial Diagnosis

**Name**: Major Depressive Disorder, Recurrent episode with psychotic features 296.34 (F33.3)

**Symptoms**:

Depressed mood most of the day as indicated by subjective report (feels sad and empty)

Feelings of worthlessness or excessive or in appropriate guilt (delusional) nearly everyday

Fatigue or loss of energy nearly everyday

Indecisiveness

Recurrent thoughts of death, recurrent suicidal ideation and suicide attempt

**Specifier:** With anxious distress (severe)

**Differential Diagnosis**: ruled out Depressive disorder due to another medical condition, with major depressive-like episodes 293.83/F 06.32, because D's general medical conditions criteria, though of clinical interest, do not predominate in her overall clinical picture of Major Depressive Disorder.

**Comorbidity:** none

**General Medical Conditions:** Diabetes mellitus and morbid obesity.

**Other Conditions That May Be a Focus of Clinical Attention:** D's late childhood/adolescent verbal and sexual abuse (trauma), attitude to long hospitalization, and concern about other family members struggling with mental illness (depression).

## Cultural Formulation

D is a Caucasian female, and this means that her parents and society expected her to measure up to a certain standard, for example, in level of education, employment, and independence. D reports feeling pressured to measure up to the expected standard due to her mental situation and slow learning. D seems to react to this situation through anger. D also reports feeling judged by God for her past actions, such as having a child out of wedlock, and perceives her present suicidal ideations and suicide attempts as the basis for rejection by God. She also reports feeling hopeless in seeing other family members struggling as she does with mental illness. This she says increases her state of despair in terms of her religious beliefs and reduces her motivation to pursue goals for wellness.

### F.  Treatment Plan

## Problems/Behavioral issues

**1). Monitor Self-Harm and Suicidal Thoughts.**

**Long-Term Goal 1:1**—following medication procedures appropriately.

**Short-Term Objective 1:1:1**—regular consultation with doctors and health care providers.

> **Therapeutic Intervention 1:1:1:1**—occupational therapy.

> **Therapeutic Intervention 1:1:1:1:2**—routine check/keeping from sharp and harmful things.

**2). Discussion on Discharge plan and follow-up for after-care plan; physical, mental, and spiritual.**

**Long-Term Goal 1:1**—Family follow-up with D's counselor and pastor to reconcile the past.

**Short-Term Objective 1:1:1**—Group process on trauma, forgiveness, and reconciliation.

> **Therapeutic Intervention 1:1:1:1**—discussion on improving D's social network
>
> **Therapeutic Intervention 1:1:1:1:2**—watch progress on D's hobbies and interests
>
> **Therapeutic Intervention 1:1:1:1:3**—journaling and periodic reviews

**3). Suicidal caution and contracting for safety**

**Long-Term Goal 1:1**—close observation/periodic spot checks day and night

**Short-Term Objective 1:1:1**—signing safety contract every two weeks

> **Therapeutic Intervention 1:1:1:1**—talk therapy for thoughts/feelings expression

**Therapeutic Intervention 1:1:1:1:2**—Family meeting to foster love and sense of belonging.

## G. SOAP note

**Subjective**—D says, "I need to let this stuff out of my chest." D is aware of how holding things without sharing or venting is affecting her. She says it feels good to share and it is relieving. D says that she is ready to engage in the long journey of change for the better, and she says she is not alone, saying. "I have my family in the journey; God is also in the journey, and they are all pushing me to do better."

**Objective**—D has her hair done, and she looks presentable. She comments that she is finding some difficulty in breathing, but she is okay without the inhaler for the moment in the session. She is getting deeper in the session and letting out details of some things that she has not shared in the past. D is able to open up more freely with less prompting in this session.

**Assessment**—D is exploring various aspects surrounding her life. She is gradually able to make connection between standing on her own and seeking support from peers and family. She is also identifying her triggers and is willing to employ coping ways in a longer period of time. She is gradually learning to be patient with herself even when she feels a bit lonely and helpless. She is learning to trust the process and to lookup for more resources for wellness in the mental, physical, and spiritual planes.

**PLAN**—I will continue to be present for D as there seems to be developing a greater therapeutic connection and help her let out more of the "stuff in her chest." I will work on plan for referral in the next couple of sessions on trauma and family therapy. I will also explore more on the insights about spiritual coping like prayer, Bible reading, forgiveness, and happiness.

## VII. Psychodynamic Formulation

A. **Initial clinical impressions** - D is very respectful and cautious in her language and mannerisms. She often appeals to her faith through mention of reading her Bible and saying her prayers. She values her spiritual exercises/activities and is always ready to discuss something about them. It appears that she is drawing some strength from her faith and is looking up to exploring it further. She is appreciative of someone listening to her, and this is instilling a sense of self-worth in a backdrop of hopelessness.

B. **Transference** - D sees me as a religious figure and projects her anger and fears of her beliefs like being punished by God for her sinful past. She also finds in me a comforting parental figure who understands and accepts her the way she is or ought to have been initially with her parents, though a feeling of closeness with parents is currently gaining ground.

C. **Counter-transference** - As I sit with D in the session, I feel like giving suggestions on religious matters or even propose a simple Bible study to flesh out some biblical issues like forgiveness she seems to be struggling with. I feel the need to refer D to someone with expertise in trauma therapy, perceiving her situation as emanating from childhood experiences.

D. **Based on answers A–C and other clinical data, other personality traits/cluster I would consider:**

Based on the many sessions I have had with D, I would consider some borderline features evidenced by unstable self-image and relationships, excessive self-criticism, and depressive mood. These features, though prominent in D, do not qualify a complete borderline personality disorder in sense of severe impairment in self and interpersonal functioning.

E. **Impact of cultural formulation on psychodynamic formulation.**

D experienced pressure and rejection at childhood and is thus seeking acceptance and love in those close to her in the moment, particularly peers and caregivers. The absence of the care she seeks or any form of trigger is reminiscent of this childhood experience and is thus contributing to her current frequent feeling of "going downhill." She is willing to make steps forward, but at the same time, she is reserved or pulled backward by the cognitive distortions that things can never be better, given the "bad past."

**F.  Psychological theories employed in engaging D and more specifically in this session.**

The theory chiefly employed is person-centered. The aspects of the person of the counselor using unconditional positive regard and being nonjudgmental are significant in restoring D's confidence in herself, which she seems to be losing in regard to expectation to win parental approval that never occurred in her situation. Through this nonjudgmental quality of relationship, D was able to share deep things in her life that as she stated has "not shared with anyone else."

# VII. Pastoral/Spiritual/Theological and Reflection Assessment

## A. Overall Clinical Spiritual Assessment

### 1. Client's current engagement with religion/spirituality/meaning-making practices:

D's spirituality remains foundational. She has a Bible, prayer book, and other spiritual books, and she has an established routine of reading and praying. She has many stories to tell about the Bible and is also knowledgeable about her faith. She also attends her church when she is well and out of the hospital.

### 2. Spiritual Assessment

D engages the scripture and asks pertinent questions. She even identifies with the characters in the Bible and especially the Wisdom of Solomon. Her sources of hope are first and foremost God to whom she prays and reads about. She is always eager to initiate a God-talk conversation and dwells on it in depth. She says that God gives her hope and encouragement when she is down. D also draws some hope, peace, and comfort from her family. She says that her family speaks with her all the time over the phone, and she loves to hear from every one of them.

## B. Theological Reflection on Current Clinical Case

**a.** There is a common theme that runs across the conversation with D, and this is explicit mention about God. Though D says that she relates with God in a personal way, prays to him all the time, and feels his presence in the Bible, she is in intense emotional pain from her reporting. She is navigating on this feeling and trusting in God, but she is confused whether God really perceives her pain. However, she is grateful that despite wishing to end her life, God is at work behind the scenes as she says, "He is the reason for why am here," meaning being alive.

**b.** D's beliefs/practices are connected to her socioeconomic/ cultural practices. She sees God as the protector and substitutes him for the missed attachment or relation she would have gained in childhood.

**c.** D's religious/spiritual practices considerably help her cope with her situation. She thus draws compassion and hope in these beliefs.

**d.** Her beliefs are helping her cope with some situations; for example, she made a reference of having suicidal thoughts in one night and counteracted that by beginning to read the Bible until she fell asleep.

**e.** Practical consequences of her beliefs include some postponement of self-harm on the belief that God will not be pleased. Remembering the family, especially her son, makes her hesitant to harm herself.

**f.** D's overall belief connects her well with God in a way that she draws a sense of hope and compassion to herself and those related to her in a very special way. She is compassionate about her mother, who is depressed, and thus she does not want to bother her. She says that she prays for her family all the time.

**g.** D's belief plays a role in how she affects others. In fact she says that she would not want anyone to feel the way she feels. She also says that she prays for and supports her colleagues in the unit as God wants.

**h.** The kind of treatment goals arising from this reflection include: incorporation of practical spiritual exercises such as composition of prayer to God on periodic/weekly basis to reflect together on the growing relationship with God and the nurturing of developing perception of God's love, forgiveness, care, and compassion; discussing the Bible and spiritual books read over the week and sharing on emerging themes; giving suggestions on biblical verses and sharing on themes such as God's protection for example in Ps. 23: "The Lord is my shepherd," "Lord, teach us how to pray,"(Lk. 11, Lord's Prayer), and Ps. 103:1-3 that says, "Bless the lord my soul, all my being bless his holy name! Bless the Lord, my soul; and do not forget his gifts, who pardons all your sins and heals all your ills,"

## C. Theological Reflection for Clinicians Growing Pastoral Awareness and Identity

**a.** The theological images that come to my mind in this session include Jesus and his mother on various occasions; for example, Mary the Mother of Jesus at the wedding feast of Cana in Galilee (Jn. 2:1–11).This closeness of Mother Mary to her Son Jesus can resonate and illumine D's closeness with her son.

**b.** The compassionate skill of attentive listening and nonjudgmental presence will make D feel accepted and welcome in the sessions and thereby form therapeutic alliances.

**c.** I feel also challenged to explore my faith more and more in a critical way, especially now that I sit with D who is struggling in her condition of mental illness and yet finds time to read the Bible and pray. I feel strengthened in my religious and spiritual exercises and activities, not only for myself but for her and others, too.

## VIII. CRITIQUE OF COUNSELING TO DATE:

D is making progress on the religious plane. However there is a lot more to be done on her childhood traumas that may be manifesting themselves in form of flashbacks and nightmares. I feel the need to explore more on this area to the point of referral for enhanced healing, forgiveness, and posttraumatic growth.

Chapter 5

# Integration: Theological and Psychological Case Analysis

## Introduction

**This section brings together the theolog-**
ical and psychological perspectives emerging from my journey

with clients as well as practical implementation of integrative

learning deemed necessary in the enhancement of therapeutic

outcomes in clinical work that is critical in pastoral clinical

mental health counseling. My learning in this field of pastoral

clinical mental health counseling and exposure to clinical work

with varied populations of people, in different settings, and

with different mental health issues have largely contributed to development of my core theological and psychological perspectives.

In my person-centered/Rogerian theoretical orientation to counseling, I found a great interplay of my theological and psychological core tenets while working especially with adult clients. In the theological plane, I intensively used the life of prayer and meditation on Word of God, belief in Trinitarian relationship, and family resilience as my foundation. In the psychological plane, I employed some of Rogers's person-centered constructs, particularly the therapeutic relationship, self-discovery for self-actualization, and active listening. The integration of these core constructs is well understood within the context of a journey with a client named D (see appendix 2 on verbatim).

D in this context was seen in sixteenth session out of the total eighteen sessions we had together within a period of eight months out of the total eleven months she spent in the hospital. There is an incorporation of brief highlights from other sessions with D, especially where it calls for elaboration of themes that run across her experiences and formulation of therapeutic goals.

## Theological Integration

The first part of analysis of the above case entails the use of theological perspectives. This is in the lenses of family resilience, Trinitarian relationship, and life of prayer as my core constructs.

Each of these constructs, as discussed earlier, have a bearing on each other. For instance, the Trinitarian relationship is viewed as family and is in a special way reached through prayer. These constructs augment well in the case of D mainly in this session.

## Holy Family and Family Resilience

In exploring the concept of family as one of my core theological constructs, I found that D was overly concerned about some of her family members' welfare, especially her mother, son, and brother who were struggling with depression as she shared in previous sessions. However, the sense of family spirit that was unfolding in our sessions was offering a sense of consolation. In my belief of family as a formidable resource in a person's overall growth, and as I related this belief with D's recourse to family in the session, I was drawn to the image of the reciprocal roles of love and communion in the family as envisaged by St. Paul regarding parents to children and vice versa (Eph. 6:1–3).

In the verbatim from C64 to C92, D shared about her members of the family, namely the dad, mom, and siblings. As she mentioned each of them, her face brightened up, and her voice assumed warm, poetic tone. Examples to illustrate this passionate or special closeness include: C65 where she referred to her one of family members saying, "She is my favorite niece" and further stated that she did not want something bad to happen with her; C73 to C82 is the mention of the core members in the family, who she passionately introduced thus: "I got my parents . . . I got my one sister . . . I got my four brothers . . . my son and my niece" Concerning all of them, she says "we are all close except one brother" (C79), whom she said did not want to have a relationship with anybody (C80). To encourage this family closeness, D got a day pass (C89) from this hospital, and as she thought of how to use it, the first thing coming to her mind was the family. She says "I will be able to meet my family again (C93) . . . I haven't seen them for eleven months (C95)." The memory of D as regards her closeness to the family reminds me of the image of a fruit tree which has different parts: flowers, leaves, branches, fruits, and trunk. Each of these parts is unique and serving individual roles and yet is interconnected with the others to make a complete whole. I empathized with D as she walked home. It reminds me of the days I was away from home and how I would look forward to meeting my family again.

At this point my mind wants to go home, having been away for the longest time in my life since leaving for studies and even now in a far-distant country. The biblical verse coming to my mind as I see a meeting point of our similar family situations in terms of longing for reunion is Psalm 133:1 (how lovely and pleasant for brothers to live in harmony).

As I reflected with D about this family closeness, I recognized growth and reconciliation of memories on her part regarding her childhood experiences and now as an adult. She said that being called "stupid" at home in her early childhood and eventually raped in late childhood (C61) that she described it "was so hard and still hurts" (C65). Yet with the spirit of family acceptance, support, empathy, and love, she was able to forgive the parents for this past sense of rejection, however difficult it had been. She is also in the path of seeking further help in dealing with the bitter experience of rape in her opening up to process the experience and resultant feelings. Though D's self-esteem was highly affected by this early experience of rejection, the present family relationship that she reported as good was positively affecting her treatment journey. In this family support she said, "I have my family in the journey (C130) . . . and being asked how the family is in her journey (T131), she said, "They push me to do better (C133)." In conclusion of sharing about family, D convincingly says, ". . . were it not for my family holding me tight, I can't" (meaning she cannot feel good for herself were it not for family support – responding to the question of feeling good about herself T141), (C141). In my belief of family as a pillar upon which basic support revolves, I see the sense of hope rekindled in D as she counts on family support. I concur with D in the holding of her family with such esteem when my mind runs back to the days of our growing up and how we would have conflicts with each other in that large family of ten, perhaps in competition of scarce resources, opportunities, and parental favor. However, as we matured into adulthood and founded our own families for majority of us, and with me taking the celibate life, we look forward to many opportunities to be together more and more though life's cares won't let us. I see this reaching out of the family through constant telephone calls and longing for a family reunion, which would be a kind of reconciliation of the past and a path to pursue for positive family relationship outcomes.

The other theological core construct running hand-in-hand with that of family is belief in the Trinity. In this respect, God is viewed as one in three persons and dwells in each Christian in a special way upon baptism in the name of the Father, Son, and Holy Spirit (Matt.28:19). This indwelling of God in the baptized individual is an incorporation into Trinitarian communion and hence entry into a special family. The concept of God and family as closely related manifests itself often in the lives of

Christians and of whom D and I are members. This was clearly pointed out in session. When I asked D about the things that are keeping her going and thus offering her a concrete sense of hope in the moment, she quickly and enthusiastically responds. She says in C141, "Right now God I mean, and were it not for my family holding me tight I can't." (meaning that she cannot find anything good about herself that would motivate her to keep going, and thanks be to God and her family offering her meaning and purpose at the moment)

## Trinitarian Relationship of Love

In course of our previous sessions, I realized that D is religious and spiritual, and I wanted to work with her around her belief as an essential resource in her treatment. That prompted me to further check on it. In this I asked directly about any other resource(s) other than family that gave her hope and meaning to life (T97), and she said in C97, "Yah, God is always on my side . . ." A discussion on faith in God and his forgiveness, and D's belief and despair come into play and unfold from C97 to

T114. D's belief that God is always on her side as just mentioned is quickly contrasted by her despair on the question of forgiveness and feeling of worthlessness. As I sat with D in this frustrating moment in the sense of her expression of doubts and desperation in forgiving herself (C98, 99, 103, 104, 105) and even losing the will to live (C115, 117), my belief in God as Trinity and thus a relationship comes into my mind. The image developing in my mind is that of Moses, after being called to confront Pharaoh, makes several complaints that he is not worthy (Ex.3:11), and that he is not eloquent (Ex.4:10). In answer to Moses' complaints, God gives timely assurance by revelation of his name, "I am who I am" (Ex. 3:14). Jesus, the son of God, also refers himself as "I am" as he says, "before Abraham was I am" (John 8:58).

This revelation of God's name as "I am" as in Jesus is transformative. It is an assuring presence, which is a loving and living one. The revelation of God as such is great though effecting gradually the transformation not only for Moses but the whole of Hebrew people as Gary and Cavins (2010) put it: "The narrative understanding for God's name is quite striking and simple: according to the logic of the story, the name Yahweh means that God is with his people. Yahweh is not a distant God but a God who is present" (p. 64).

D appeared to have reached a dead end, but God was present and she acknowledges this though she feels burdened by the past difficult experiences and the present struggle with mental illness. She confessed a sense of hope hidden in God—hidden amid all these. In the situations D is facing, I am reminded of what Dr. Houck (2009) said, relating to role of God in human suffering and the search for meaning: "Indeed, no matter what we face, whether intense suffering or the intense longing for God in that spiritual desert, there will be times when the clouds part, springs of water will flow, and a night spent in tears will lead to joy in the morning" (p. 146).

**Life of Prayer and Meditation on the Word of God.**The last core theological construct that I have used in this encounter with D is prayer. D opened this idea of prayer by explicitly stating in C97 that "God is on my side. I pray to him at all times." As I listen to D say this, I am reflecting on the personal relationship D is expressing with her God. It seems to me that prayer for D is something she is accustomed to as she states this with ease and conviction. However, the look on her face and a long pause that followed the statement left me wondering. This brought me to ask the probing question in T98, checking out what she tells God in her prayer. In response she said she seeks forgiveness from God but as per what she has done in the past, it is difficult to experience this forgiveness and her guilt overcomes her (C98–99). This is especially so when as she recounts what she was told by a person of a different faith tradition that God cannot forgive everything.

As a priest and pastoral counselor, knowing the depth of religious beliefs in meaning-making in our lives, I walked D through exploration of her beliefs, including faith tradition, religious affiliation and the subject of prayer, knowledge of the Bible, and God's forgiveness (T100–113, C100–114). I am impressed to see D grow and discover the things she wants to pray for, which God may forgive. In the course of the conversation, my role is that of a priest, who upholds prayer and forgiveness. I am impressed to see D grow and discover the things she wants to pray for which God may forgive. These things she enumerates as having a child out of wedlock (C108) and being able to forgive herself (C110).

## Psychological Integration

In the psychological perspectives of my journey with D, I drew a lot of insight from my person-centered Rogerian theoretical approach. With Rogers (1980) as the lead guide in my approach, I was able to see D as a person endowed with capacity for growth as he writes:

> Individuals have within themselves vast resources for self-understanding and for altering their self-concepts, basic attitudes, and self-directed behavior; these resources can be tapped if a definable climate of facilitative psychological attitudes can be provided. (p. 115)

The mention of psychological attitudes in this statement by Rogers points to me D's psychological disposition. Newman (2009) reminds us that as relates to psychological system: "emotion, memory, perception, problem solving, language, symbolic abilities and our orientation to the future all require the use of psychological processes" (p. 6).

## Therapeutic Relationship

The first of the application of my psychological core concepts in this person-centered Rogerian approach is therapeutic relationship. This concept sets in right away in the beginning of this session with D as our connection is now well established, this being the sixteenth session of individual encounter. We also had many more other encounters in group settings within the eight-month span of my internship in this hospital.

In the opening of this session, D easily and freely shares her feelings of the moment, stating that she is upset by two things: first is the change from the unit where she has spent most of her time (C2–6) and, second, linked to this is her discomfort with a peer roommate who tried to harm her (C8–24). Some of the concepts emerging in this relationship include those of trust and openness (C2–24). When D shares these feelings of the moment with me, I see through her eye contact and facial expression what she expresses, and I let her take the lead as I make minimal verbal interactions (T2, 4, 5, 6, 9, 10, 11 . . .). Most importantly, communicating powerfully in nonverbal way included pauses, eye contact, and so forth (T3, 4, 5, 7, 8, 9, 10).

This minimal interaction, but with active listening, on my part keeps in mind Rogers's way of unconditional positive regard to the client in which therapist accepts each individual and lets the client be what he or she is in the moment. This allows what Rogers (1980) calls "whatever immediate feeling is going on—confusion, resentment, fear, anger, courage, love, or pride" (p. 116). As I sit with D, I let her know that what she feels is okay, and I create this environment with a nonjudgmental attitude expressed through open questions.

An example of this was in the introductory part of the session where she complained about the change of unit and the relationship with roommate. She reported that as the situation escalated, the roommate was transferred to another room, though within the same unit (C8–18). Within the flow of this event, my intervention is limited only to short responses of "okay, eh, and pauses (T10–20), and she freely shared and expressed her feelings. Based on our earlier sessions and processing of feelings, I see a progression on part of D in creating a safe space for herself in this session as evidenced by clearing of a grudge she had earlier with a colleague who had thrown away her plants, and with whom she now reports as having made up (C27–28).

Another instance in which I used the caring or unconditional positive regard was the concern about D's physical wellbeing in this session. She said that she had not used her inhaler (C41–45), and I asked about her comfort and safety in her breathing (T42–47) at which she said she will be all right.

What I see as a special breakthrough in this relationship is D's sharing about being raped at age 12 (C117). She admitted that this made her hate life and further said she has not been able to open up even to the family (C125) as much as she trusts in them(C127). The unfolding of the session seems to have made her feel that in our relationship that honors trust, acceptance, and safety so that she can share to the point of saying that she wants to engage in a positive journey of growth from the painful past, trusting her counselor(T128/C128), her family (C130), and God (C133). D with a bright face exclaimed, "That is why am still here!" (C134)and further said, "I see myself moving forward" (C136).

## Self-Discovery for Self-Actualization

The second psychological perspective I employ in this session is self-discovery for self-actualization. Rogers (1961) believed that individuals are hindered from the discovery of their true selves by layers that pile up over the years. He states: "To remove a mask which you had thought was part of your real self can be deeply disturbing experience; yet, when there is freedom to think and feel and be, the individual moves toward such a goal" (p. 110).

In the session, D and I navigated around the search for her true identity through her experiences and especially the part of herself she feels difficult to share. These include her being raped at age 12, being called stupid when younger (C61), and the consequence of hating life from that moment (C117). D concluded the session by pointing to her loneliness (C145) and pointing out that she hears voices (C146–154) especially telling her that she is a failure (C150). As a counter technique to end the negative voices, she focuses on that which she likes to think: her niece (C156) whom she refers as the favorite niece (C65). D also mentions her son and the niece as having a special place in her heart (C82), and she draws some hope in thinking about them. In an earlier session, D said that she postponed self-harm due to a thought about her son, and she said, "I got to be there for him."

## Active Listening

The final of my psychological perspectives is active listening. This shows itself through my clarifications (T29, T57), while making D reflect back on her own feelings of the moment as she shares the story or incidences about herself (T31, T42, T59). I also check on how our sitting together in the session feels to her as she shares such confidential experiences (T69, 129).

D feels that she has been heard and therefore goes deeper in the session to share the above difficult experience that she has not shared with anyone else. As she said in C124, "I have not been able to open up . . . some part of me does want to (C127).

Being actively listened to (T129), not only in words but being able to clarify and communicate back this experience, makes D feel set in motion from where she had been stuck. And she brightened up, she said, "I see myself moving forward" (C136).

## Conclusion

As I conclude this chapter, I look back and see clearly the interplay of my theological and psychological core concepts relating in a tremendous way to produce great results. I have been impressed to hear empowering words coming from D's mouth with a force pointing to change, growth, and transformation. In C25 she reports having cleared a grudge that she had before, though was hard to do.

Another very important discovery on D's side is the fact that she feels and sees herself moving forward, saying, "I see myself moving forward (C136) . . . is Scary (C137) . . . because I hate change, and I have to accept it" (138). She crowns this by saying, "I am not alone in the journey for I have my family and God (C141), I read the Bible, color, talk (C143), and do other readings.

It is quite fulfilling on my part to realize that along this long journey and many sessions, there is a restful outcome and our common belief in Jesus. It gives me courage to believe in words of Jesus who says, "Come to me all you who labor and are overburdened and I will give you rest . . . my yoke is easy and my burden light" (Mt. 11:25–30).

D had been in this hospital for a good period of time, and she let me know she was ready for discharge in the next couple of weeks. She said that she was ready for the next move, which was a half-way home she would stay in before eventually getting back home. The journey of eight months' encounter with D in individual as well as group sessions in this hospital provided a good framework and a basis to look back and forth in putting together a toolbox for D. As we looked forward to the termination of the session, D and I went through the goals we had been formulating and checked out what had been accomplished and what needed further exploration.

Our work at that point was made easier given the periodical summaries that we had been evaluating together. Looking back on this journey with D, and now in the termination stage of our session, I was deeply moved by her resilience and dignity as compared to her entry into this journey. It was also inspiring on my part to hear D state some of the outcomes of engaging in this individual counseling. Some of these as she reports are: starting to write her memoirs, updating her journal, and being present for her aging parents as well as seeing her son together with nephews and nieces safely growing to adulthood. This last outcome on consciousness of the role of D as a mother reminded me of the greater responsibility of single parents as Emery (2004) recounts:

> Interest in single-parent families and their influence on children stems both from the increased occurrence of these households and from evidence that youth in these homes may be exposed to numerous environmental stressors that place them at risk for subsequent poor outcomes. (p. 1)

## Chapter 6
# DISCERNMENT

**The feeling of the journey, as I engaged in** this work from experience in Neumann University and as I furthered the integration of my learning in pastoral counseling with practical applications, is that of rising sun that spells beginning of a new day. It does indeed occur to me that what I searched for in those many days before coming to Neumann has finally been achieved. As I stated in the introduction about my experience with various groups and populations of the people I worked with previously, the question of wanting to offer a deeper response particularly to the challenges of life posed by many always recurred. The search drove me to undertake many courses in addition to the intense priestly formation and these studies have complemented what I already knew and yielded a comprehensive understanding of pertinent tenets in the pastoral counseling field as laid out in this book.

Another major discovery, which has manifested itself in a more concrete way in the process of this work is the journey of self-discovery. In course of the study, research, and practical work, there was always the greatest room left or rather dedicated to response of the question "Who am I? As a counselor, the question points out to personal strengths, challenges, and areas for improvement. Intentionally engaging especially the growing edges, resolving the past otherwise underlying issues, and committing to open ongoing formation to the person of the counselor one is called to be is not always easy. A challenge of one's beliefs and even learning to be comfortable to engage someone with beliefs and values contrary to your own and offering yourself to tolerate such vulnerability was initially hard. It requires competence of counselor educators and a great practice, motivated by the nature of counseling as a special helping relationship. Such has been my take in the course of study though openness to ongoing learning for enhanced competencies, professionalism, and collaboration is called for.

The long journey in the program and looking back to its culmination gives me courage to re-echo that there are indeed *Refreshing Fountains on the Pilgrimage.* One who sows seeds looks forward to their germination and growth. The sower projects that, given the conducive environment and provision of all that is needed, the desired results are possible. However, there arises situations that project contrary results, and the sower who does not distant himself from the process is able to make necessary interventions in due time. This reminds me of Joseph (Gen. 41:37–49) who in his wisdom consulted with Pharaoh on the coming dry spell and laid plans ahead to secure plenty. And guess what? With timely interventions, those periods of famine were never felt by those people and their animals. It is valuable to compare the situation of the sower to that of Joseph.

The counselor and the client in the session trust in the process together and accomplish tasks that have power to inform, form, and transform not only the client but both of them in different levels and to a great extent. I wish to recall as I conclude some of the Franciscan values that characterize learning in my *alma mater* Neumann University: Catholic education in Franciscan tradition. The core values are contained in the acronym RISES. As espoused therein, "Neumann *rises* on the values of Respect, Integrity, Service, Excellence, and Stewardship" (Office of Mission and Ministry 2011, p. 7). These values are not only relevant to the counseling program but unifying factor in entire University—Neumann Community. I take with myself these and many more values as an alumnus of the Neumann community and in the family of pastoral counselors and church ministers.

I feel empowered in mind and spirit with enthusiasm, hoping to implement my learning and practice among all the people I encounter, particularly people of Africa and my native country of Kenya and anywhere else God wants me. Like Mary Mother of God, I humbly say: "May it be done to me according to God's will" (Lk. 1:38).

# REFERENCES

American Psychiatric Association. (2013). Diagnostic and statistical manual of mental disorders: DSM-5. Washington, D.C: American Psychiatric Association.

Benedict XVI, Pope (Joseph Ratzinger), (2006) *Jesus of Nazareth,* New York: Doubleday.

Calloway, D., Gaitley, M., Hahn, S., Kelly, M., Martin, C., Richards, L., and Wuerl, D. (2015). "Introduction: An Invitation to Mercy." In *Beautiful Mercy.* (p. 11). Erlanger, KY: The Dynamic Catholic Institute.

Deal, P. J. and Magyar-Russell, G. (2015). "Religious and Spiritual Assessment in Pastoral Counseling." *Understand Pastoral Counseling.* Maynard, E. A. and Snodgrass, J. L. (Eds.). New York, NY: Springer Publication Company

Emery, R. E. (2004). "Single-Parent Families: Risks, Resilience, and Change." In M. Coleman and L. Ganong (Eds.), *Handbook of Contemporary Families: Considering the Past, Contemplating the Future*. Thousand Oaks, CA: Sage Publications. Retrieved from http://ezproxy.neumann. edu/login?qurl=http%3A%2F%2Fsearch.credoreference. com%2Fcontent%2Fentry%2Fsagecontfa%2Fsingle_ parent_families_risks_resilience_and_change%2F0

Fowler, J. W. (2000). *Becoming Adult, Becoming Christian: Adult Development and Christian Faith*. San Francisco, CA: Jossey-Bass.

Gary, T. and Cavins, J., (2010).*Walking with God: A Journey through the Bible*. West Chester Pennsylvania: Ascension Press.

Houck, J. (2009). *The Apostle Peter: His Words Should Be Red Too*. Aston, PA: Xulon Press.

Hunter J.R., Malony H.N, Mills L.O., Patton J., (Eds) (1990), *Dictionary of Pastoral Care and Counseling*. Nashville,TN: Abingdon Press.

Julian of Speyer (1999)."The Divine Office of Saint Francis."
In Armstrong R.J., Hellmann J.A.W., andShort W. J. (Eds).
*Francis of Assisi: The Saint* (p. 336), Hyde Park, NY: New
City Press.

Justes, E. J. (2006). *Hearing Beyond the Words: How to Become
a Listening Pastor.* Nashville, TN: Abingdon Press.

Kornfeld, M. (2012). *Cultivating Wholeness: A Guide to Care
and Counseling in Faith Communities.* New York, NY:
Continuum International Publishing Group.

Lartey, E. Y. (2003). *In Living Color: An Intercultural Approach
to Pastoral Care and Counseling.* Philadelphia, PA: Jessica
Kingsley Publishers.

Merton, T. (1971). *Bread in the Wilderness.* Collegeville, MN:
Liturgical Press.

Newman, Barbara M., and Newman, Philip R. (10thed.) (2009)
*Development through Life: A Psychosocial Approach:
Groups Process and Practice.* Belmont, CA:Wardsworth
Cengage Learning.

Rogers, C. (1957). "The Necessary and Sufficient Conditions of Therapeutic Personality Change "University of Chicago. (Reprint of an original work published in 1957) *Journal of Consulting Psychology,* Vol. 21, pp. 95–103. Retrieved on 4/3/2015 from: http//www.shorline.edu/dchris/psych236/ Documents?Rogers.pdf.

Rogers, C. (1961). *On Becoming a Person.* Boston, MA: Houghton Mifflin Company.

Rogers, C. (1980). *A Way of Being.* Boston, MA: Houghton Mifflin Company.

Rogers, C. (1980). *Carl Rogers on Encounter Groups.* NY: : Harper and Row.

Rogers, C. and Farson, R., (1987). Active Listening*: Communication in Business Today.* Newman, R.G., Danzinger, M.A., Cohen M., (eds). Washington, DC: Heath and Company.

Six, J-F. (1998*). Light of the Night: The Last Eighteen Months in the Life of Therese of Liseux.* Notre Dame, IN: University of Notre Dame Press.

Walsh, F. (2009). *Spiritual Resources in Family Therapy*. New York, NY: The Guilford Press.

Yalom, D. Irvin (2009). *The Gift of Therapy*. New York, NY: Harper Perennial Publishers.

Office of Mission and Ministry (2011) *Catholic Education in the Franciscan Tradition*. Aston: PA, Neumann University Press.

# VERBATIM

T = Therapist (Pastoral Counselor)    C = Client (Counselee)

T1: How are you today?

C1: I am doing okay, I guess. [PAUSE]

T2: eh

C2: A little upset . . . but . . . yah [PAUSE]

T3: I hear you say that you are a little bit upset; would you talk more about that? [PAUSE]

C3: They moved my unit.

T4: eh. [PAUSE]

C4: I hate change.

T5: Okay. . . [PAUSE]

T6: So . . . that change made you a little bit upset.

C5: Yes.

T7: Okay. . . [PAUSE] . . .

T8: And . . . how are you feeling about that change? . . . [PAUSE]

C6: Oh, I don't know.

T9: eh . . . [PAUSE] And . . . within that change and the new environment are there some things that you feel that . . . you are not comfortable about . . . or that make you feel upset? [PAUSE]

C7: Oh yah . . . [PAUSE]

T10: eh . . . [PAUSE]. What about those things?

C8: One is we're on the same unit—a girl that I don't like,

T11: Okay,

C9: And just don't hear,

T12: Eh,

C10: That just doesn't make it easier,

T13: Eh,

C11: may cause a lot more. [PAUSE]

T14: Eh . . . [PAUSE] Is there any other thing related to that.

C12: Not really.

T15: Not really . . . [PAUSE] . . . How are you finding that . . . you say . . . that there is someone you feel uncomfortable with in the unit?

C13: Oh yah.

T16: How does that, eh . . . how does it feel to you?

C14: Oh, we had to set exact boundaries . . . [PAUSE] . . . so .
. . though finally she scolds me. [PAUSE]

T17: She was . . . you said she was bothering you?

C15: Yes, she was my old roommate.

T18: Okay. The roommate. Okay. . . [PAUSE] are there some
things you felt not comfortable with?

C16: Yah. She tried to harm me.

T19: Harm you?

C17: Yah . . . Then they moved her.

T20: Okay.

C18: But we are on the same unit that she is . . . [PAUSE]

T21: Okay, this was before . . . when did you move to this unit?

C19: When did I move to this unit?

T22: Yes.

C20: Today.

T23: And previously you said the experience was previous . . .
some other time?

C21: Room in the unit next door.

T24: Okay. [PAUSE] . . . is the situation is now settled.

C22: Oh yah

T25: But you are not with the same person in the unit, I mean in the room.

C23: yah . . . [PAUSE]

T26: I hope that gives you a little settling of the mind. Or are there some things that you feel are still not cleared about that?

C24: Yes.

T27: Okay.

C25: I already cleared upon the grudge I had.

T28: Eh . . .

C26: Like today yesterday. I know it was hard to do . . . [PAUSE]

T29: What did you say was that grudge . . . what was it?

C27: Against a guy named R. He threw a couple of my plants. I kept grudge for a couple of days, but I felt finally will hurt me in the long run.

T30: Eh.

C28: So me and him made up yesterday.

T31: Ah. How did you feel when you made up after those few days of staying in the grudge?

C29: It felt embarrassing.

T32: Felt embarrassing?

C30: Yes. Because I never apologize . . . This was so deeper .
. . [PAUSE]

T33: It sounds like there was someone who was kind of mediating the process for you to apologize . . .

C31: Yes I was wrong.

T34: Eh.

C32: Yes. I was wrong.

T35: You take it to yourself that you were wrong.

C33: Yah.

T36: Say more about that.

C34: [PAUSE] I talked to N, nurse N, because I had difficulty breathing . . . like I feel right now. Then she called R for me to apologize to him . . . It was very embarrassing, for I knew I was wrong.

T37: You knew you were wrong.

C35: Yes.

T38: and that was why was kind of embarrassing for you to apologize.

C36: yah [PAUSE]

T39: Eh, and what was . . . what did the other person do after you apologized?

C37: He said him and I have a problem between us.

T40: Okay.

C38: but he has his own . . .

T41: It looks like the person did not know how you felt after that, and that's why I think he said he did not realize there was something between you.

C39: Yah.

[PAUSE]

T42: You also said that you are running kind of short of breath, and you are also feeling the same now.

C40: Yes.

T43: How is it right now?

C41: I didn't put my inhaler.

T44: Oh, you use your inhaler?

C42: Yah.

T45: Okay. Are you comfortable and safe when we are here with you?

C43: I will be okay.

T46: Okay. Your breathing is alright?

C44: A little bit.

T47: A little bit, okay. [PAUSE] So, is that something that would bother you in this session?

C45: Not really.

T48: Okay. [PAUSE] . . . What else would you want to talk about today?

C46: I don't know. [PAUSE]

T49: How are you going on with your treatment and your journey?

C47: I have been to here at [Belmont] for eleven months.

T50: Eleven months!

C48: I came here March the sixth last year.

T51: So from March last year . . .

C49: I have come a long way.

T52: Is a long way.

C50: Yah, there is still a lot to be done, but . . . is a long way.

T53: How is that long journey of eleven months being here . . . what does it look like to you?

C51: It doesn't look promising, like when I see people come and going . . . and am not with them . . . at same time sounds scary to leave here . . . [PAUSE]

T54: How are you feeling . . . to see people come and leave, some few days, few months, few weeks, they leave you here?

C52: It sounds scary to leave here . . . [PAUSE]

T55: It sounds scary for you to leave here. A period of . . . eleven months is definitely . . . a good duration of time . . . I believe you have been able to . . . eh, know all the corners and the many things about the place.

C53: Yah.

T56: What are some of your memories of being here for eleven months?

C54: Was okay, but I knew I needed help, but as time went, and I left here June of last year, went for a program, I tried to commit suicide, and they brought me back here the end of June . . . [PAUSE] I have been here ten months and one month in that other place but all together is eleven months.

T57: I now get it clearly that there was a time that you had a break in the month of June.

C55: Yes.

T58: You went to that program.

C56: Yes.

T59: You also said that in that program you had suicidal thoughts.

C57: Oh, no, I attempted it.

T60: Oh, Okay. I get it.

C58: Yah.

T61: You attempted to commit suicide . . . [PAUSE] What kind of things went on between getting out of here and going there? Is there something related to that transition that made you attempt suicide.

C59: Yah, I hate change . . . [PAUSE] I usually go downhill when change happens . . . [PAUSE]

T62: So you say you hate change, and you go downhill when change happens. . . . [PAUSE] Are there some situations in your life you have experienced such changes that have made you go downhill, and what are some of these that you can remember?

C60: There is too much to remember . . . [PAUSE]

T63: What are some of the things you can remember, one or two events or episodes that maybe you can remember that made you go downhill?

C61: Being called stupid when I was younger . . . and at twelve I was raped. So a lot went downhill then . . . [PAUSE]

T64: I hear you, and I hear about the situation you encountered at that early age . . . [PAUSE] Do you see . . . were there . . . from the moment you were called stupid when you were growing up, being raped, . . . how does that feel today, maybe this moment as we talk?

C62: Was so hard.

T65: Was so hard . . . it still hurts . . .

C63: Yah.

T66: Have you been able to seek some help or someone journeying with you along that . . . [PAUSE] . . . Are there some situations or ways in which this has been addressed . . . Do you . . . or have you addressed it in a situation like this, therapy . . . or through other help may be spiritual . . . or any setting?

C64: Only through flashback of it.

T67: Flashback . . .

C65: Yah, when my niece turned 12, I still have flashbacks, because she is my favorite niece, and I don't want her to . . . [PAUSE]

T68: So when she turned that age, you kind of remembered what happened to you at that age.

C66: Yes . . . [PAUSE]

T69: What do you feel when you tell me this story . . . this experience?

C67: And I have not told any of my family members . . .

T70: You have never told to any of your family members.

C68: Yes.

T71: That is why I say whatever we share here is confidential and meant for your own benefit as you share it out . . . How do you feel when you share out this?

C69: I feel okay. I mean I need to get this stuff out of my chest.

T72: Okay. . . [PAUSE]. When you let it out of your chest and speak it out is a kind of relieve—is that what you mean?

C70: Yah . . . [PAUSE]

T73: What are some of your coping ways that help you as much as you have this experience and some flashbacks keeping on coming? Are there some ways that you try to look at it in a way that kind of gives you some hope to move on . . . [PAUSE] Are there some coping ways?

C71: I have been coloring and drawing; that keeps me busy than thinking about other things.

T74: What are other things that you do?

C72: I have been trying to call my parents, but no one answers the phone.

T75: Who are your family members?

C73: I got my parents,

T76: Both of them are living?

C74: Yah, but divorced.

T77: Okay.

C75: I got my one sister,

T78: eh.

C76: I got my four brothers.

T79: Four brothers. Are there some other members close to you in the family?

C79: We are all close except one brother,

T80: Eh.

C80: He doesn't want anybody.

T81: It sounds like when you call them, you get some hope, and that is why you would like to get in touch with them . . .

C81: Yes . . . [PAUSE]

T82: What are some of the sources of your hope, what gives you hope and keeps you moving day by day?

C82: It is literally my son and my niece . . . [PAUSE]

T83: Okay.

C83: and my sister puts it that I can't help myself no more.

T84: Eh.

C84: Because I want to be there when my niece graduates school and go to college. . . .

T85: So she says that you cannot help yourself and do things for yourself?

C85: yah.

T86: What makes her say this to you?

C86: Because she doesn't want me see my niece no more.

T87: So she is the mother of your niece?

C87. Yah.

T88: Sounds like you have a good relationship with your niece?

C88: Yah.

T89: How is that like? Do you do things together or what makes it like that?

C89: I used to take her to do things, but when I am in and out of hospital, I don't do much . . . [PAUSE] That is why I got a day pass. I got to find a way when I can use it.

T90: What is that again . . . ?

C90: Day pass to leave the hospital.

T91: Oh, day pass, I get it now . . . so you have one?

C91: Yah.

T92: Okay.

C92: I have to find a way to use it, sometime next week.

T93: So you will be able to meet her . . .

C93: I will be able to meet my family again; they cannot be able to come here.

T94: Is there a rule that they cannot come here?

C94: Well, they live in Delaware County.

T95: Oh, because of distance.

C95: I haven't seen them for eleven months . . . [PAUSE]

T96: That sounds a long time.

C96: Yah.

T97: What else would you want to talk about? . . . [PAUSE] I hear you say the family gives you hope, your niece . . . is there anyone else or higher power . . .

C97: Yah, God is always on my side. I pray to him all the time . . . [PAUSE]

T98: As you pray to God, and as you relate with him, what do you tell him? Would you want to share how?

C98: How he forgives me all my sins. I always tell him that what I have done wrong. I can't take the guilt any more.

T99: Okay. . .

C99: He is supposed to forgive everything, but I heard from Jehovah Witnesses one come from my door one time and used to talk about God and told me that only sin God does not forgive is having a child out of wedlock. And I know I had a son out of wedlock, so that kind of hurts. So even if I trust in God, I went down a little bit.

T100: And before you met a Jehovah Witness, or rather, what is your religious affiliation? . . . [PAUSE] Do you go to a certain church or certain faith . . .?

C100: I go to Baptist church.

T101: You belong to Baptist church. . . You were brought up in that Baptist church?

C101: Yes.

T102: How is your practice to date?

C102: Is okay. I mean, I read the Bible and . . . [PAUSE]

T103: When you say that God forgives everything, or is supposed to forgive all, what makes you feel that he does not forgive you for your child out of wedlock?

C103: Because I do everything wrong. Yah, I don't expect him to forgive me everything.

T104: And when you say from your statement that God forgives everything, how do you find that you being part of everything that God forgives . . . [PAUSE]How do you see yourself fitting in his forgiveness?

C104: I see myself bothering . . .

T105: Eh . . .

C105: I know God forgives everything . . . but down there I don't know what to do.

T106: It sounds like this area of forgiveness you would want to learn more about . . . [PAUSE] You say God forgives everything but has not forgiven you . . . [PAUSE] And what does the Bible say when you read the Bible about forgiveness?

C106: I have to read it again. [PAUSE]

T107: And in the Bible there is prayer of our Father. Do you recite this prayer . . . Do you know it?

C107: Our Father who art in heaven.

T108: Yes. And there is a part in that prayer that says, forgive us our trespasses as we forgive those who trespass against us . . . [PAUSE] Are there part of things in your life that you want God forgive?

C108: I want him forgive for having a son out of wedlock. But sounds when I was pregnant this was something hard to forgive . . . [PAUSE]

T109: Is there anything else you feel that you would ask forgiveness of God?

C109: For my own . . .

T110: Your own . . .

C110: My own being able to forgive.

T111: Your own forgiveness?

C111: I don't know to forgive myself. I know to forgive everybody else, but I don't know how to forgive myself.

T112: I think this is a huge revelation. I mean to be able to forgive others is something great, to begin to forgive others and to forgive ourselves. . . . [PAUSE]

C112: Yah.

T113: What are the things that you need to begin to forgive yourself?

C113: I don't know . . . [PAUSE]

T114: As you have told me, you would want to work on forgiving yourself.

C114: Because I know am always wrong . . . [PAUSE] I believe every breath I take is wrong.

T115: You mean . . . every . . . by breath you mean every move . . . Say more about that . . .

C115: No, every breath I make is wrong. I am tired of living. I think I should be dead . . . Yah.

T116: What makes you think that way?

C116: I have always thought that way since I was a child.

T117: Are there some things that you can remember made you think that way?

C117: I just hated life for long time . . . [PAUSE] All what happened to me when I was age twelve; I mean . . . made me hate life.

T118: I hear what you say. Of the event that happened when you were twelve . . . [PAUSE] What do you mean when you were twelve, and what happened to you when you were twelve?

C118: I was raped . . . [PAUSE] And I believe it was my fault.

T119: You believe it was your fault . . .

C119: Yah

T120: Yes.

C120: Yes.

T121: What makes you believe it was your fault?

C121: I knew better. I knew what is right and wrong.

T122: When you were twelve?

C122: Yah.

T123: As you say when we are that age (12), we know what is right and wrong. At the same time we are growing up. A twelve-year-old much as still is a child has knowledge but has a lot more to learn. And that is I think why until one is eighteen is not yet able to make a meaningful decision . . . And that age is still tender age. At the same time I hear what you say, that what could be done when one is young memories could still be living with the person.

C123: Yah.

T124: And I see what you say about it. So is there anything that can be done in our sessions and with other people who are helping you in your journey for example inside this facility here or outside? Do you have some resources that can help you process that?

C124. I have not been able to open up, though.

T125: You have not been able to open up.

C125: Yah.

T126: Okay. What would make you open up?

C126: Oh, I don't know. Some part of me doesn't want to.

T127: Some part of you doesn't want to. Are there some people you trust in a way that you can be able to pour out your soul and your experience?

C127: I trust my family, but I don't know right now. I don't want them to know everything in the world. [PAUSE]

T128: And as you keep opening yourself in the treatment and in your journey, I believe there are people trained and able to listen to you and eventually journey with you to process this experience and therefore be able to get through and be able to get the growth out of that. Some events happen in our lives, and they are so deep and they rob us of our personality, of our esteem, our dignity and they really put us so down. And as you say that you trust God,

[C: nods the head saying, "Oh, Yah"] . . . [T: continues] as a resource, there is a growth that can come in the letting go. That is not a one day process, is a journey . . . [PAUSE].

C128: Yah.

T129: How do you feel when I talk to you about the journey . . . would you want to engage in such a journey?

C129: Is a long journey.

T130: Is a long journey. Do you think of positive aspects of engaging in such a journey until something positive is born.

C130: Yah. I have my family in the journey.

T131: How is your family in the journey?

C131: They push me to do better.

T132: Eh. I see something positive. I think now I relate what you said about your family and how they are wishing good to you.[PAUSE] (C nodes her head, T continues . . . so your family is on that end.

C132: Yah.

T133: And what else is on that end pushing you to . . .

C133: God is on my end; I think he is pushing me to do better too.

T134: Eh.

C134: That's why am still here.

T135: And I see that you are also in a place that is offering that . . . Do you see it happening in your life?

C135: I am trying to get out of the place.

T136: Yah, but in a place that eventually will make you realize this journey you are making and to team up with the family and God . . . What about yourself in the journey?

C136: I see myself moving forward.

T137: How is this moving forward?

C137: Is scary.

T138: Is scary, what is scaring?

C138: Because I hate change, and I have to accept it.

T139: Do you mean the change in the positive journey that you are making?

C139: Yah.

T140: What is that change looking like to you?

C140: Positive. I got things to achieve for myself, and I see it working.

T141: Let me ask you a few things before we conclude . . . [PAUSE] What are some of the things that you feel good about yourself for the moment?

C141: Right now God I mean, and were it not for my family holding me tight, I can't(feel good about myself)

T142: God and your family.

C142: Yah

T143: Are there some exercises or activities that you do, that make you feel better? You talked about coloring, reading . . . are there others? [PAUSE]

C143: Talking.

T144: Talking. As we conclude, is there anything that you would want to talk about in this moment?

C144: Not really.

T145: So you do not have any question . . . I just want to tell you that I am there, in case you feel you would want to talk about your journey and also that in this facility there are people trained and who would be willing to support you in your journey and that you are not alone . . .

C145: (interjects in a soft voice) I feel alone.

T146: (reflects back gently) feeling alone. Do you want to say something about it, in a minute before we conclude?

C146: Feeling alone and talking to myself.

T147: Do you talk to yourself?

C147: Yes.

T148: And what do you tell yourself or what is the conversation?

C148: I hear voices, I mean.

T149: Eh, you hear voices . . . within yourself?

C149: Yes. I try to avoid to, but it's hard to do.

T150: Next session we shall talk about that, unless there is something specific you want to talk about the voices . . . Do you hear them as we talk now?

C150: They keep telling me that I am a failure.

T151: They keep telling you that you are a failure.

C151: Yes, and I can't make it in life.

T152: Do you focus on the other sources of your hope? As you said God is here and that is why you are still living. Do you give the voices the chance to let you feel that you are a failure or would you want to see yourself in another . . .?

C152: I believe my voices.

T153: What makes you believe them?

C153: Because I believe all the negative things I hear.

T154: When you believe all negative things that you hear, what comes of your life? What does it turn to be?

C154: It goes downhill.

T155: When it goes down, what happens?

C155: I tell myself to back up.

T156: How do you do this?

C156: I do this by thinking about my niece.

T157: So you have a way of coping not to go down and you focus on something else.

C157: Yah

T158: As we conclude, do you have any question or concern or something else to say?

C158: No. I can't focus on something else right now.

T159: We are going to end our session. Whatever we discuss remains confidential and what you have shared as I reflect it back to you, there are situations that make you go down and as you look at some of the resources that surround you, will be able to draw some hope and something to make you move on. And in case you have any other question or concern . . . am here and will really appreciate to listen to you. Thank you very much.

C159: Thank you.

# PSALM 23

The Lord is my Shepherd;

there is nothing I lack.

In green pastures he makes me lie down;

to still waters he leads me;

he restores my soul.

He guides me along right paths

for the sake of his name.

Even though I walk through the valley of the shadow of death,

I will fear no evil, for you are with me;

your rod and your staff comfort me.

You set a table before me

in front of my enemies;

You anoint my head with oil;

my cup overflows.

Indeed, goodness and mercy will pursue me

all the days of my life;

I will dwell in the house of the LORD

for endless days.

# PRAYER

Lord Jesus Christ, Son of the living God, in union with the Holy

Spirit, come to us!

We all belong to you for you have created us,

And you have called us by our names, as you called your apostles.

Help us to respond to your call everyday,

and let us call others to follow you in the same way.

Everyday is a great gift from you,

and a special moment to experience your love and goodness.

Lord Jesus Christ, Son of the living God,

in union with the Holy Spirit, be in us!

Let us be in you as you are in us.

Let us bring others to you that they may experience your love.

May we in union with you be bound together with an ever-lasting cord.

Let us surround your table, taste your goodness, and go forth proclaiming:

"The Spirit of the Lord is upon me,

Because he has anointed me

to bring glad tidings to the poor.

He has sent me to proclaim liberty to the captives

and recovery of sight to the blind, to let the oppressed go free,

and to proclaim a year acceptable to the Lord." (Lk. 4:18,19)

# Group Process Sketch

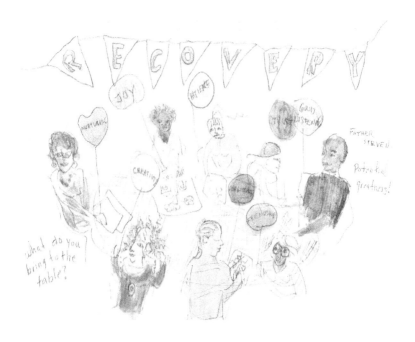

# Thoughts and Action Control Exercise

**S**TOP

Don't react

**T**AKE A BREATH

Slow and controlled

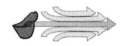

**O**BSERVE

What am I thinking?

What am I reacting to?

What emotions am I feeling?

What am I feeling in my body?

**P**UT THINGS IN PERSPECTIVE:

Are my thoughts fact or opinion?

What are my clues that the thought is true?

Can I find clues that it might not be true?

How can I argue against the thought?

What would I tell a friend in the same situation?

**P**ROBLEM-SOLVE & PRACTICE WHAT WORKS

What is the best thing to do for me, for others, for the situation?

What will the consequences be for my actions?

What are the pros and cons of my actions?

Will my actions help me achieve my goals?

# Pictorials

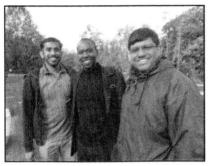

*Left: Colleagues in life help support your journey.*
*Bottom left: Praying the rosary gives hope and confidence.*
*Bottom right: Community celebrations give joy and strength.*

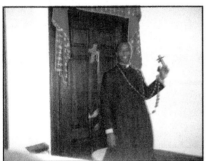

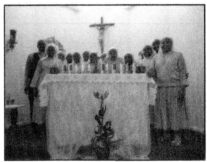

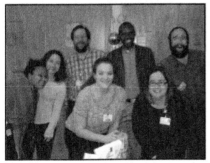

*Left: Teamwork builds success.*
*Bottom left: Mentoring the young ones.*
*Bottom right: Enjoying good company with a good show.*

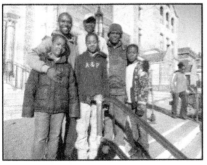

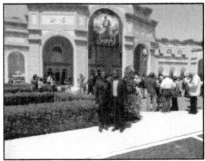

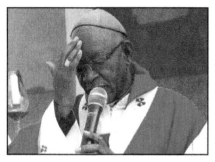

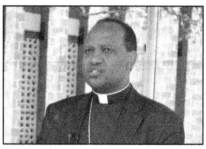

*Upper left, upper right, right: Church leaders praying, encouraging, and supporting the people of God.*

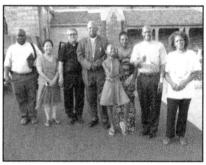

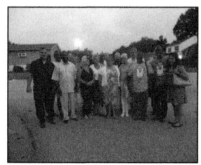

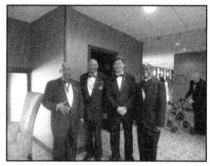

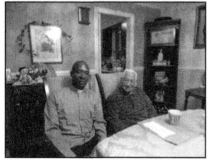

*Upper left: Enjoying together on a cool, summer night. Upper right: Belonging to a group gives a sense of support. Left: Listening to the wise words of a senior colleague.*

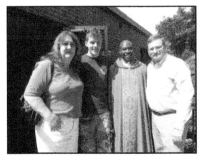

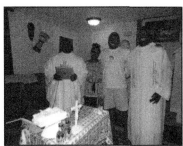

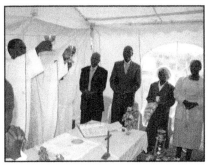

*Upper left, upper right, left:*
*A family that prays together,*
*stays together.*

*Right, lower left, lower right:*
*Raising our hearts and minds*
*to God in prayer keeps the*
*Church united and her members*
*nourished*

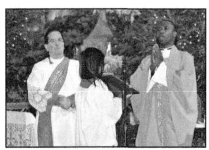

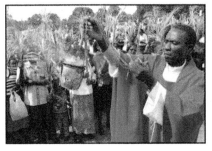

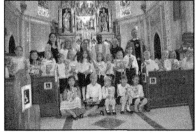

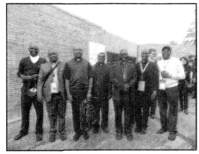
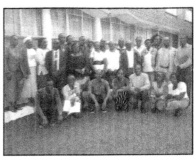
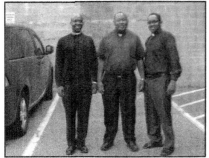
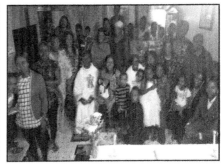
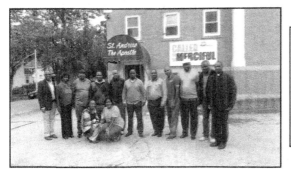

*All: Church as a family, in prayer and pilgrimage.*

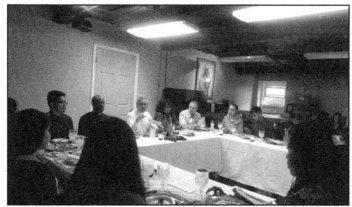

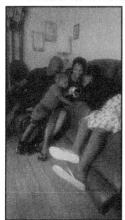

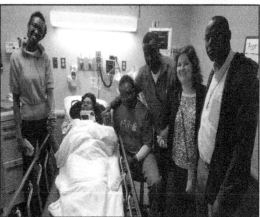

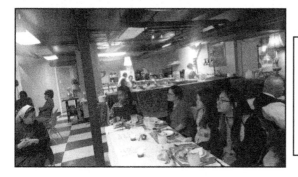

*All: Family living together in joy in all circumstances.*

141

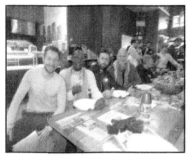

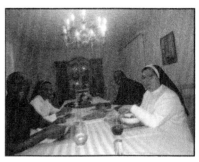

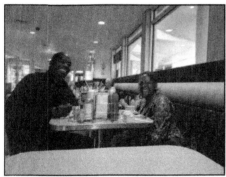

*All: Sharing
and refreshing
in joy
and gratitude*

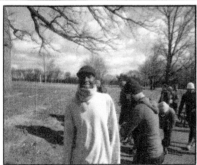

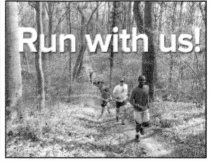

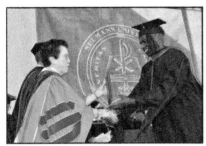

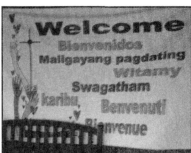

*All: Welcome
to the world
of learning
and sharing
with others.*

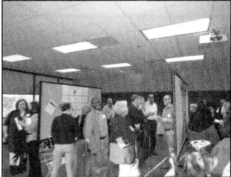

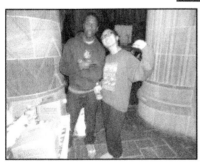

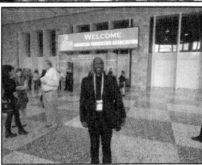

CPSIA information can be obtained
at www.ICGtesting.com
Printed in the USA
BVOW10s1452090917
494413BV00003B/3/P